Helping
Women
Recover
FROM
Abortion

Nancy Michels

Helping Women Recover

FROM

Abortion

Nancy Michels

BETHANY HOUSE PUBLISHERS

MINNEAPOLIS, MINNESOTA 55438

A Division of Bethany Fellowship, Inc.

Published by Bethany House Publishers
A Division of Bethany Fellowship, Inc.
6820 Auto Club Road, Minneapolis, Minnesota 55438

Printed in the United States of America

Library of Congress Cataloging-in-Publication Data

Michels, Nancy.
    Helping women recover from abortion / Nancy Michels.
        p.   cm.
    Bibliography: p.
    1. Abortion—Religious aspects—Christianity. 2. Abortion counsel-
ing—United States. 3. Pastoral counseling—United States. 4. Abortion—United States—Psychological aspects. I. Title.
HQ767.25.M54 1988
241'.6976—dc 19   88–10447
                                                     CIP

ISBN 0–87123–621–4 (pbk.)

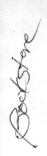

To my mother, Edna Michels,
and to all mothers.

NANCY MICHELS has a wide-ranging background in writing. She has done extensive editorial work with Better Homes and Gardens Books, has been the Public Relations Director and Communications Manager of the Better Homes and Gardens Real Estate Service, and has been a Communications Specialist for Blue Cross and Blue Shield of Iowa. Her experience related to the abortion issue comes from her involvement with Lutherans for Life. She and her husband make their home in Davenport, Iowa, and they have three children.

ENDORSEMENTS

"*Helping Women Recover From Abortion* is a poignant documentary of the pain-filled lives of many aborted women. It is essential reading for those who think that abortion is a solution to unplanned pregnancy and for those who would counsel the growing sisterhood of permanently scarred women. *Helping Women Recover From Abortion* reveals the hidden horror of abortion *and* the healing help that is available."

Dr. Jean Staker Garton
Author of *Who Broke the Baby?*
and nationally known pro-life leader.

"Parents are parents forever, even of a dead unborn child. Nancy Michels' book is an important acknowledgment of this psychological reality and the trauma that is abortion. Many women and men who have experienced abortion, as well as many counselors, will find this book invaluable on the difficult journey from grief to healing."

Vincent M. Rue, Ph.D.
Executive Director of the Sir Thomas More Marriage and Family Clinic.

ACKNOWLEDGMENTS

Many people have made this book possible, especially Nathan Unseth and Carol Johnson of Bethany House Publishers. Their concern for the women who suffer from Post Abortion Syndrome, as well as their patience, are deeply appreciated.

And the women—and men—who shared their abortion experiences with me—thank you for your willingness to relive the painful memories so that others will better understand just what a woman suffers *after* the abortion.

I also am indebted to all the professionals whose research and clinical counseling give credibility to the reality of Post Abortion Syndrome.

Finally, I wish to thank my husband, Tom, who supports my concern for all hurting people. His patience and understanding are my strength.

TABLE OF CONTENTS

CHAPTER ONE

WHY WOMEN HAVE ABORTIONS

Jennifer flipped through the magazine, the words and articles racing by too quickly to be read. She tossed the magazine onto the rest of the unread pile and checked her watch. "Two and a half hours!" she muttered to herself. "How long does it take to get the results of one pregnancy test?"

She looked up anxiously as the door to the examining area opened. "Jennifer," the woman said, "would you come in please?"

Jennifer slid her purse under her arm and stood. "Well?"

The woman said nothing but led her to a small office. Jennifer sat in a chair opposite a roundish woman. She assumed her name was Lois by the name plaque on the desk.

Lois leaned forward in her chair, studying Jennifer's face. "Your test was positive."

Without warning, the tears Jennifer had been holding back for days suddenly spilled out. It felt like someone had slugged her in the stomach. After several minutes,

Jennifer looked up from her tears to find the woman silently watching her.

"I'm so ashamed," she said haltingly. "I should have known better. I'm no kid. I'm 22."

Lois nodded her head, but said nothing.

"The father doesn't care; my family will be humiliated. I can't take care of a baby all by myself." Jennifer put her hands to her face and wept harder. She reached for a tissue from the box on Lois's desk. After blowing her nose, she went on. "I guess I have to have an abortion."

Lois spoke softly. "We don't do abortions here. But I can refer you to a clinic. Would you like me to set up an appointment?"

Jennifer bit her lip and rubbed her thumbnail on the corner of the desk. "I guess so. I don't really have any other choice, do I?"

"It doesn't sound like it."

Ten minutes later, Jennifer left the office, a small paper tucked inside her purse. Monday, 2:00 p.m., was all it said.

She walked down the street, wishing she had someone to talk to. Wishing someone would come up with a better option. But what other options were there? Her heart raced in fear. *Abortion.*

If she talked to her parents, what would they say? They had divorced three years earlier. Jennifer tossed her head a little to get the wind-blown hair out of her eyes. *Dad wouldn't care. Mom and her new husband would probably find some way to give the baby up for adoption.*

Jennifer shook her head. Adoption would never be an option. A friend had given her baby up for adoption. Her grief and pain never seemed to end.

Jennifer turned the corner and wandered into a park. She sat on an old bench near the children's playground. As the kids fought and played, shrieked and cried, she realized she could never raise a child alone.

I'm doing the right thing, she thought. *Abortion is really my only option.*

As the next five days crept by, Jennifer shut out the doubts she had about the abortion, and focused on the rightness of her choice. She wouldn't have to worry about upsetting her parents. She knew the baby's father didn't care. He had only been a one-time fling. A fling to fill an aching, confused heart. She never would have had the fling either if she hadn't let her inhibitions slip away with her use of marijuana that night. No, pregnancy should be a choice made between two people who intend to spend a lifetime together.

Monday dawned a beautiful morning. Jennifer wished it would go away. Her stomach cramped with fear and nerves. As she climbed aboard the bus for the 20-minute ride to the clinic, she wondered if anyone would know her destination. She wondered if anyone cared.

At the clinic, Jennifer wished she were having a bad dream and would soon wake up. She flipped through more magazines until the attendant called her name.

Again, she sat across a desk, this time from another woman. This one explained the abortion procedure, then read a list of the possible side effects of abortion. Her voice sounded much like a tape recorder.

"Wait!" Jennifer said suddenly. "What was that you said about sterility?"

"Just a formality," the woman said with a smile. She leaned across the desk and patted her arm. "You needn't worry. We are required by law to read this, but it doesn't happen very often."

Confused and afraid, Jennifer didn't know if she wanted to go through with the abortion.

The woman sensed her hesitation. "Oh, go ahead and sign it. There's really nothing to worry about."

Jennifer didn't want to sign the paper, but she felt backed into a corner with no other choice.

After more waiting, the attendant led Jennifer to a small, clean room. "Here, put this on," the attendant said, then left, closing the door behind her.

Jennifer put on the thin, paper examining gown and a pair of paper slippers. The attendant returned with a paper cup for a urine sample. She also drew blood from Jennifer's arm.

Soon Jennifer was alone again, with only her thoughts and the sounds of people scurrying back and forth outside her door to keep her company.

Her breath came heavier and faster, tears waiting just beneath the surface. She ran to the door and flung it open. "Won't you please talk to me?" she cried to a passing nurse.

"What's wrong? Are you afraid?" the nurse asked as she came in the room.

"I . . . I don't know if I am or not." Jennifer looked into the eyes of the nurse. "This is wrong. I know abortion is killing, and I don't want to be here."

"No one wants to be here," the nurse replied. "Everyone is scared. Don't worry. It will be okay."

Soon after the nurse left, the doctor came in, followed by his assistant. He washed his hands, ominously silent, while fear and doubt filled Jennifer's mind.

Then pain replaced the fear and doubt. Strong and steady pain. The assistant explained that the doctor was dilating her cervix. The pain came because the cervix was not ready to be dilated.

Jennifer watched flashes of metal as the doctor grabbed one rod after another, each graduated in size.

"It hurts, it hurts!" Jennifer cried out.

The room filled with a deafening whir as the suction machine came on. Jennifer gulped in large amounts of air.

"I can't bear it," she whispered to the assistant, who stroked her hair and held her hand. A buzzing noise grew louder inside her head as Jennifer began to pass out.

Without a word, the doctor completed his procedure, covered the suction machine with a towel, and wheeled it away.

After Jennifer dressed, a nurse led her to the lounge area. She nibbled on toast and sipped tea, not really feeling like nourishment, but knowing that her shaky body needed something to stabilize it.

Inside, she felt empty, stripped of her own self-respect. The words, "I've killed my baby," pounded through her mind. It seemed absurd that physically she could look so well when her inner self had been so beaten and hurt.

As she left, the nurse stopped her. She put her hand kindly on Jennifer's arm. "Now wasn't that easy?"

Sadly, Jennifer nodded. "Yes, it was. Yes, it was."

Years later, Jennifer realized that if one person had told her not to have the abortion, she wouldn't have done it. "Abortion was available and real accessible. I told the people at the clinic my fears, but they never offered any alternatives. All I could think of was abortion. I couldn't really see beyond the moment."

Many women like Jennifer, who've had abortions, will admit they really didn't want to resort to abortion, but they did so because it seemed the only alternative to an unwanted pregnancy. Even if they considered other options, they did not receive support from friends, relatives, or counselors. At that time they also did not have the emotional strength to investigate other options on their own. Abortion was offered as the easy solution. As Jennifer said, "It was so accessible."

If many women don't want to resort to abortion, then why do they do so? What reasons lie behind their choices?

Are these reasons valid? In this chapter, we will examine the more common reasons why women choose abortion and illustrate them with real-life experiences. To these women, the reasons were strong and real enough to overcome any thoughts of abortion as wrong or the taking of a human life. In some cases, the reasons were based on fear and emotional instability, while others were founded on financial concerns and the need to maintain a lifestyle that did not include raising a child.

"I didn't know it was a baby."

Sandi had three abortions by the time she was 22 years old. "I viewed being pregnant as an inconvenience. I dropped out of school and had received no education on fetal development. I never felt abortion was wrong." When Sandi turned 31, she was confronted with the reality of what she had done. She viewed an abortion film at her church and saw the fetal models on display. "The fact that I had killed three children hit me hard. I started crying and wondered where those models were when I was in the abortion clinic."

A woman faced with an unwanted pregnancy will often deny that the child developing inside her womb is a human being. Her doctor might call it "a product of conception." Someone else might say, "It's just a blob of tissue." Both descriptions deny personhood to the child.

There is no law that says a pregnant woman must be informed of her baby's development before she is allowed to have an abortion. Few women will search for this information on their own.

Most abortions are performed during the 18th week of pregnancy. It is at this age that the unborn child's body is completely formed, including fingerprints. Just 2 weeks earlier, at 10 weeks, the unborn child has a discernible heartbeat (the heart has been beating for 1 month), and brain waves have been measurable for 2 weeks. Also at 8 weeks, a baby feels pain, responds to touch, sucks her thumb, swims naturally, and will grasp an object in her palm. After the 12th week, nothing new develops within the child's body. All the parts are there on a miniature scale; they just get bigger and stronger.[1]

Because she can't see her baby, a woman with an un-wanted pregnancy rationalizes that she really isn't carrying a human being. She will convince herself that an abortion is the solution to an unpleasant problem, not ending a life.

"I didn't think of it as a baby; it was just the condition of being pregnant," said Jane, who at 21 had the first of her two abortions. Although both her parents knew about the abortion, her father never talked to her about it. "I was being treated like I had a rare disease. When the cause of it was taken away, I would be back to normal."

"I was so ashamed."

Maureen grew up in a middle-class Catholic family and attended an all-girl parochial school where she was voted "Most Mary-like" by her senior class. An honor student, Maureen felt expected to graduate from college and make something of herself. Her self-image changed when she found that she was pregnant a month before her April wedding. "I couldn't tell my parents I was pregnant and shatter their image of me," Maureen said. "Also, an older sister had had to get married and I didn't want people saying that about me. I panicked. After the abortion, I couldn't get out of bed to go to class in the morning. I felt joyless and thought that I was a terrible person. My wedding lost all of its meaning."

---

[1]Tract, *8-Week-Old-Developing Baby* (Hayes Publishing Co., Inc., 1984.)

The image of a good Catholic girl who waits until marriage to become sexually active was shattered. Maureen had to learn how to live with this new self-image, one she never imagined she would have.

Becoming pregnant, whether a woman is married or unmarried, betrays her active sexuality. If she is unmarried, she feels she has been caught; all of her friends and relatives will know she is sexually active. So, if she can "terminate the pregnancy" before it's obvious, no one will know she was pregnant or even had a sexual relationship.

A young girl who is sexually active may deny her activity, but a pregnancy forces her to face reality. Only an abortion will allow the thought process "I'm living by the rules" to continue and prevent an unwanted confrontation with parents or other authority figures. While a teenager may be ashamed of becoming pregnant today, it's usually because she got "caught" at being sexually active, not because of the pregnancy itself.

"My mother pressured me into having an abortion."

Unplanned pregnancies aren't unique to unmarried teens. In fact, one-fourth of the 1.5 million abortions performed in the United States every year are effected on married women.[2] Often these women are also pressured into having an abortion by either their parents or their husband. Perhaps the woman is in a bad marriage and her parents wish she would leave her husband, and, possibly, return home. They fear that if she has a baby, she will stay in the marriage.

Husbands may encourage an abortion if they feel they cannot financially afford another child. Some want their

---

[2]Dr. and Mr. J. C. Willke, *Abortion Questions & Answers* (Cincinnati, Ohio: Hayes Publishing Co., Inc., 1985), p. 81.

wife to work outside the home without the distraction of childbearing and childrearing.

Nancyjo's husband walked out on her and her two small children when she was five months' pregnant. Her mother told her she'd better have an abortion, because, "No man is ever going to want you with three children, let alone the two you already have."

Within hours of her husband's leaving, Nancyjo went to a doctor who told her that because of her advanced pregnancy, she would have to have the abortion that very day. Still suffering from the shock of her husband leaving and without time to think about what she planned to do, Nancyjo checked into the hospital and proceeded with a saline abortion.

Her fear that she had done something terribly wrong was confirmed when Nancyjo delivered her perfectly formed daughter herself early the next morning, after twelve hours of painful labor. The nurses didn't arrive until after the dead baby was delivered. Nancyjo held her child and saw that, yes, she really was a person, with a full head of dark hair and perfect, but tiny, fingers and toes.

Nancyjo was devastated by what she had allowed to happen. "I killed her, I killed her" pounded through her head. Her heart ached for her dead child, but her overpowering guilt for what she had done wouldn't let her grieve and it soon controlled her life.

"My boyfriend said I had to."

At 15, Louise had the first of her two abortions. She didn't want to have the abortion, but fear and shame kept her from telling her mother about the pregnancy. Then the father of the baby threatened to end their relationship if she didn't have an abortion.

"When told I was pregnant," Louise said, "I immediately thought, 'I have to get an abortion.' My boyfriend had said I would have to.

"I knew it was wrong to have the abortion. Before the abortion, I would talk to the baby and cry, telling it I didn't want to do it. But I knew I had to because I didn't want to lose my boyfriend.

"He went with me to have it done and waited in the waiting room. But afterwards he forgot about it. I was bitter and really angry at what he had made me do. We broke up six months later."

Pressure to abort may come from the father of the child, whether or not the couple is married. If they are unmarried, he may encourage abortion to avoid marriage or the responsibility of financial support for the child. He will also support abortion to avoid telling his parents that he is the father of a child.

In other cases, the father of the child may truly be concerned about the mother's welfare and reputation. He feels responsible for the pregnancy and may not want his girlfriend to suffer through the likely turmoil that a baby would cause in her life. He is willing to pay for the abortion, perhaps even go with the woman to the abortion clinic, to fulfill his obligation to make things "the way they were."

While some parents may not protest their son's sexual activity, they certainly would object to him getting a girl pregnant. As long as they can't be sure of his sexual activity, they don't have to say anything; but once there is proof (a pregnancy), they can't deny his involvement. So they will encourage abortion to avoid public knowledge of their son's sexual activity and the resultant embarrassment.

If the couple is married, the father of the child may encourage abortion for financial reasons. Perhaps extended unemployment has eroded feelings of being able to support another dependent.

If the couple is older, the husband may not want his wife to endure the hardship of pregnancy and labor, only to be burdened with the responsibility of raising a child for the next 18 years.

In their later years, it is an embarrassment for both the father and mother to admit to the mother's pregnancy, especially if their other children are grown. In an age when birth control is readily available, married couples are expected to plan their family and not encounter any "surprises."

At 40, Charlotte became pregnant with her third child. At first, she thought it was menopause because of her irregular period and frequent fatigue. But a physical exam revealed her eight-week pregnancy. Her husband, Frank, was as surprised as Charlotte to learn of the pregnancy. The younger of their two children, a senior in high school, would soon be off to college. Charlotte had received her nursing degree the previous year and now enjoyed her career as a surgical nurse. Frank didn't like the thought of her raising another child. Proud of her career and appreciating their second income, he looked forward to building a nest egg for their retirement.

"Frank suggested the abortion, and I went along with him," Charlotte said. "I really didn't want to go through a pregnancy at my age and give up my career or try to juggle a career with motherhood. I felt I had sacrificed enough of my life."

"My doctor said the baby was deformed."

A doctor may strongly recommend an abortion if the unborn child has a physical defect. Through ultrasound testing and amniocentesis, doctors are better able to determine if the unborn child has any physical and mental disabilities in the very early months of pregnancy. Parents are faced with the decision of whether or not to abort their child if any of numerous possible defects are found, from heart problems to Down's syndrome. The mother may want to go ahead with the pregnancy and do everything possible to correct the problem, but the father may not want to bear the financial responsibility for the necessary surgeries. For him, it would be easier to abort the baby and try again.

The shame of giving birth to a defective child is a key factor in a couple's decision to have an abortion. In today's society, perfection, even in the children we bear, is expected. We're told not to settle for anything less. So if we can determine that an unborn child is less than perfect, we are not condemned for killing it. Rather, we are expected to.

Susan and Roger had tried to have a baby for six years. Susan eventually conceived with the aid of fertility drugs. During her 16th week of pregnancy, an amniocentesis disclosed the baby had Down's syndrome. The doctor recommended aborting the fetus, but Susan wasn't sure. Roger could only visualize long years of caring for a handicapped child and the limitations placed on their lives as a result.

"I didn't want to see our marriage ruined over a deformed baby that didn't have to be born. I figured it would be an act of kindness not to allow the fetus to develop," he said.

Sometimes a woman is counseled to abort a fetus when she has previously given birth to handicapped children. She may not want to risk giving birth to yet another handicapped child, especially when the available tests cannot determine if the child will suffer from birth defects.

Such was the case with Marie. Her premature daughter

was blinded at birth and her premature son was afflicted with hyaline membrane disease. When pregnant for the third time, she asked her doctor to perform an abortion. Since this occurred before abortion was legal, her doctor refused her request. Marie didn't pursue the issue and gave birth to a healthy son just one week before his due date. She thanks God that she didn't abort a healthy infant.[3]

"This isn't a good time for a baby."

After postponing her college education for eight years, Becky enrolled in a local college. She planned to have a career as a certified public accountant before she was 34 years old. She and Jim had struggled long enough on one paycheck that never seemed to cover all their needs. Now that their two daughters attended school, she felt free to pursue her dream.

A month before the beginning of classes, Becky learned she was pregnant. "I was devastated. And afraid. I knew if I told Jim, he would make me cancel my school plans and I didn't want to do that. I had waited too long to put my plans on hold for another five years," said Becky. "So I had an abortion and never told Jim. It just wasn't a good time to have a baby."

If one asked a group of pregnant women if this was a good time for them to have their baby, it is likely that most of them would say no. In our minds, the best time is when we are financially secure and in a stable environment, preferably between the ages of 25 and 35. But few women conceive when it is the "best time." And few know when the best time really is. Lives change every day and no one can plan for certain that "best time" to have a baby.

---

[3]Anonymous, "All Life Is Priceless," *Pentecostal Evangel* (July 27, 1986), pp. 12–13.

A woman who discovers she is pregnant when she wasn't trying to conceive needs time to adjust to the news, whether she's happily married and financially secure or unmarried and living alone. Just being pregnant is a change in lifestyle.

While most women don't go to their first prenatal exam desiring an abortion, it can be an option offered to them. A standard question asked by obstetricians/gynecologists is, "Was this pregnancy planned?" If it wasn't, they may offer the option of performing an abortion themselves or refer the woman to another doctor. Some doctors will ask, "Do you want to terminate this pregnancy?"

Even if they don't mention abortion or the option of terminating the pregnancy, the doctors could plant this possibility in the minds of women by simply asking if the pregnancy was planned.

Many women considering abortion can't see beyond problems the pregnancy would create. They may see "baby" but only in red capital letters underlined and followed by exclamation points. They think of the demands of the baby and child affecting their lives. They don't award their developing child any positive qualities: companionship, intelligence, athletic ability. To some women, having a baby is something to which you have a negative reaction.

Michigan Judge Randall Heckman in his book *Justice for the Unborn* tells us: "Our society professes to love children, but, with legalized abortion, it should be clear that this love is very conditional and shallow. . . . This anti-child attitude does not expressly hate children to the point of wanting to kill them. Rather, it is more subtle. It says: Children are an inconvenience to my lifestyle now. Children are an excessive expense and a pain to raise. They prevent me from realizing my potential. For the good of my family and myself, I want my children to be planned. Since I am now pregnant with an unplanned child, I should take steps to end my pregnancy."[4]

Couples who have more than two children may find themselves the objects of cutting remarks and crude jokes. Ruth and Gary had the perfect family: a boy and a girl. When Ruth became pregnant with her third child, people would say to her, "But you already have a boy and a girl. Why would you want to get pregnant again?"

In our society, if a couple has two boys or two girls, then it's acceptable for them to try for a third child of the opposite sex. Other than that, many people have difficulty understanding why anyone would want to raise more than two children today. We have conditioned ourselves to have the perfect life, which includes cutting down the number of acceptable offspring to two or less.

Mothers of two children are now finding themselves faced with society's disapproval if they are responsible for an "unplanned" pregnancy. They may want to have the baby, but they fear what other people will say. They may also feel the financial pressure of providing their children with all the material desires that society says parents owe their children. One more child may make it impossible for them to afford everything for all their children, and they do not want to deny their older children any conveniences or luxuries. Abortion seems to be the most likely answer.

"My doctor made it sound so easy."

Women considering abortion are often not told what actually happens during the abortion procedure or the possible physical side effects of abortion. *The abortionist is neither required to discuss the abortion procedure he*

---

[4]Randall J. Heckman, *Justice for the Unborn* (Ann Arbor, Mich.: Servant Books, 1984), p. 142.

will use nor to disclose the physical effects of abortion.

In the case of Nancyjo, her doctor told her, "I'm going to take a little fluid out and put a little fluid in. You'll experience severe cramping and that will be it." He didn't tell her she would have to suffer through 12 hours of labor or face physical risks that ultimately left her infertile.

A doctor may say that he must offer abortion as an option if a woman is pregnant, whether or not she indicates she wants one. He does this to protect himself from a possible lawsuit if the child is born physically or mentally handicapped. However, there is no law that says he *must* discuss abortion as an option.

A doctor may honestly believe that he is helping the woman when he offers abortion as an alternative to an unplanned pregnancy. He may indeed be making life easier for her at that moment, but he is not being totally honest about the procedure when he does not disclose the physical and emotional effects the woman will suffer as a result of the abortion.

"My pastor said it was up to me."

If a woman considering abortion belongs to an organized church, she may decide to seek her pastor's counsel. She may want to know what the Bible says about abortion, or, she may hope that the pastor will tell her that abortion is morally wrong and is not an option.

Such was the case with Karen, a 30-year-old divorced mother of two small children. Karen had been a church member all her life and was raised to believe that life is a gift from God. But she felt it wouldn't be right for her to have another baby, especially when she wasn't married to the father. She didn't know if she would ever marry again, after a divorce that had left her wary of lifelong commitments. She could probably afford the financial costs of the pregnancy and raising another child, but she doubted she would have the emotional energy to be a mother to three children. Her career as an attorney demanded much of her life.

Karen decided to consult her pastor about what Scripture says regarding abortion. To her surprise, her pastor acted uncomfortable when she discussed the abortion with him in his office.

"You know, Karen, this really is a personal decision, something that only you can decide," he said. "Of course, the church will support you in whatever you choose."

Karen left his office totally confused. Why couldn't he just say abortion is either right or wrong? How was she supposed to know if it was right in her situation?

Unfortunately, many organized churches have no policy or biblical position on abortion. They leave it up to each pastor to counsel their parishioners as they see fit. Few pastors feel equipped to counsel anyone about abortion. When women come to them for counseling, they try to be compassionate and look at the situation from the woman's viewpoint and how she will be affected by motherhood. They tend to ignore the real issue: whether killing an unborn child, for any reason, is sanctioned by God. They want to help the woman but, in the process, ignore the child.

"My counselor said abortion was the only answer."

As a high school senior, Julie learned that she was pregnant. She attempted to investigate other options besides abortion. "The counselor at the social service organization didn't have any answers for me. She made it seem so hopeless, even thinking about having the baby. 'Look what you're throwing away,' she told me. She tried to make my future look so bleak," Julie said. So Julie did what the counselor suggested and proceeded to have the abortion.

A woman with an unplanned pregnancy is under much stress and is not likely to make a rational decision about keeping or terminating her pregnancy. She is at the mercy of the people she seeks for advice. In many cases, she is looking for help, but not necessarily help to get an abortion.

In Julie's case, she wanted a place where she could live until the birth of her baby and then either relinquish it for adoption or keep it. But her counselor kept reminding her how a full-term pregnancy would hinder her college plans and her lifestyle. She didn't help Julie see beyond the immediate future.

Of the women interviewed for this book, none had the experience of receiving counseling that looked at options other than abortion when faced with an unplanned pregnancy. Rather, the counselors seemed to be abortion facilitators, who were there to promote abortion, particularly at the facility they represented. Perhaps they believed they were really helping the women solve a difficult situation with the quick solution that abortion offers.

In the next chapter we will consider the emotional effects of abortion and the price women pay for the "solution" that abortion offers.

CHAPTER TWO

THE EMOTIONAL
EFFECTS OF ABORTION

For many women, their first emotion after having an abortion is immediate relief—that is, relief that they are no longer burdened with an unwanted pregnancy.

Mona said, "I felt that now I could put things back together again, even though I was sad that it couldn't be different."

Research has shown that feelings of immediate relief are shortlived and are soon replaced by guilt, sadness, and regret. Although Mona felt relief that her problem had been solved, she also felt sad that she had the abortion. Later, anger replaced her relief: anger at the circumstances that led to the abortion, anger at her lover for getting her pregnant, and anger that when she divorced her husband and married her lover, he had a vasectomy. Now she will never bear his child. But mostly, Mona is angry with herself for, as she said, "not being a stronger person and going through with the pregnancy."

To cope with her anger, Mona suppresses thoughts of the baby she aborted. "I don't let myself be a part of the

29

past. I don't think about it. I just want to get things back to normal."

To avoid emotional pain, Mona rationalized her abortion by telling herself that she had no other choice. She feared losing her two children by her first husband if he found out she was pregnant by another man. She admits to herself that she wanted the baby, yet felt it wasn't the right time, so she had no choice but to abort. Also, she feared her parents' reaction. They had not been supportive of her when a pregnancy led to her first marriage. "They were terrible to me and made me feel like I was a bad person. It took years to get over that night [when she told her parents]. Whenever I thought of it I would get sick physically. That's why I felt I had no choice about my abortion. I couldn't possibly tell them I was pregnant by another man."

The guilt, anger, and fear that Mona has experienced are all common emotional reactions to abortion. In fact, they are just a few of the more common reactions now identified in Post Abortion Syndrome (PAS), the condition that occurs when women repress the grief that results from the loss of their aborted child. PAS is a valid syndrome characterized by distinct patterns of symptoms that may be diagnosed as "post traumatic stress disorder," officially recognized by the American Psychiatric Association in 1980.[1] Other emotional reactions that a woman suffering from PAS might experience include depression, grief, anxiety, sadness, shame, helplessness, hopelessness, sorrow, lowered self-esteem, distrust, hostility toward self and others, regret, insomnia, recurring dreams, nightmares, anniversary reactions, suicidal behavior, alcohol and/or chemical dependencies, sexual dysfunction,

---

[1]Dr. Vincent M. Rue, "Post Abortion Syndrome," presented at Healing Visions, the First National Conference on Post Abortion Counseling, University of Notre Dame (August 11, 1986), pp. 32–33.

insecurity, numbness, painful re-experiencing of the abortion, relationship disruption, communication impairment, isolation, fetal fantasies, self-condemnation, flashbacks, uncontrollable weeping, eating disorders, preoccupation, distorted thinking, bitterness, and a sense of loss and emptiness.[2]

What are the factors of PAS?

There are five factors or criteria that identify a woman suffering from PAS:[3]

First, the woman will have experienced the stressor event, that is, the abortion itself. This would include occurrences leading up to the abortion, the abortion procedure, and the feelings the woman experienced as she aborted. This would also include emotions she felt during the decision-making process of whether to have an abortion and the responses she may have received from the principal people in her life (parents, counselors, pastors, friends).

Second, the woman re-experiences the abortion in at least one of the following ways: recurrent memories of the abortion or the unborn child, recurrent dreams about the abortion or unborn child, and the sudden feeling as if the abortion were reoccurring. In the latter case, she may see herself lying on the procedure table and watch as the abortionist vacuums or suctions her baby out through the tube. The terror and pain she felt during the abortion will be as

[2]Dr. Vincent M. Rue, "Current Status and Trends in the Study of Post Abortion Syndrome," presented at Healing Visions II, the Second National Conference on Post Abortion Counseling, University of Notre Dame (July 19, 1987), available on tape from the National Youth Pro-Life Coalition Educational Foundation, Jackson Avenue, Hastings-on-Hudson, NY 10706.

[3]Dr. Vincent M. Rue, "Post Abortion Syndrome," presented at Healing Visions, the First National Conference on Post Abortion Counseling, University of Notre Dame (August 11, 1986), p. 36.

real in her mind as it was the day of the abortion.

Third, the woman experiences an avoidance phenomena—that is, she is less involved with her external world in at least one of the following areas: a marked diminished interest in her personal life, a sense of detachment from others, a reduced ability to feel or express emotions, depression, less communication and/or increased hostile interactions. Mona said, "I feel as if I'm a colder person now. I'm numb when I had been so vulnerable before. I used to grieve for dead babies or hurt children. Now there is nothing."

Fourth, the woman will experience at least two of these associated symptoms: hyperalertness, exaggerated startle reaction or explosive hostile outbursts; sleep disturbance; an increase in the severity of the symptoms when she is reminded of the abortion (such as seeing or hearing about pregnant mothers, and exposure to nurseries or clinics); guilt about surviving when the unborn child did not, guilt about the abortion decision-making to resolve the problem pregnancy, and the inability to forgive herself for her involvement; memory impairment or trouble concentrating; and avoidance of activities that remind her of the abortion.

Fifth, the woman can be categorized according to one of three PAS groups: those stressed (either acutely or chronically), those not stressed, or those not currently stressed but who are at risk due to a delayed reaction.

A woman is acutely stressed when the stress occurs within six months of the abortion experience and lasts less than six months. Loss of interest in people and events in her personal life is typical. She may be less communicative and more depressed.[4]

The woman is chronically stressed when the syn-

4Ibid., p. 37.

drome lasts longer than six months. This phase is characterized by irritability, startle reactions, and unwelcome remembering, either conscious or unconscious, of the abortion.[5]

The PAS reaction is termed delayed when it occurs more than six months after the abortion event. The typical time for this phase to appear is seven or eight years after the abortion. In the delayed reaction, denial is used heavily, and there is a growing emotional numbness and distraction with everyday matters.[6]

How a woman reacts to her abortion and her level of PAS are determined by three factors: biological (what actually happened in the abortion procedure), psychological (her set of moral values), and spiritual (moral and religious questions she must answer about her action). Also, her previous experiences that reveal her history of stress and the environment she returns to post-abortion will help determine her emotional reaction to this traumatic event.[7]

How many women suffer from PAS?

Some PAS clinicians will say that every woman who has an abortion will suffer from PAS to some degree. While that may be true, we can determine a more conservative number based on the same percentage used to estimate the number of Vietnam veterans who suffer from post-traumatic stress disorder. The figures vary from 500,000 (17%) to as many as 1,500,000 (50%) out of 3 million veterans who served in the Vietnam War. With more than 1.5 million abortions occurring annually over

---

[5]Ibid., p. 37.
[6]Ibid., p. 37.
[7]Terry L. Selby, M.S.W., "Post-Abortion Counseling Techniques," presented at Healing Visions, the First National Conference on Post Abortion Counseling, University of Notre Dame (August 12, 1986).

the past 15 years, it is estimated that there are nearly 12 million women who have experienced an abortion. Applying the 17 percent incidence rate used on the veterans, we find that more than 2 million women suffer or are at risk of suffering from PAS. Using the 50 percent incidence rate, that figure could be as high as 6 million women.[8] This is a substantial number of hurting women.

Again, not all women who have had abortions suffer from PAS. Those who do will find that the degrees of suffering vary. But for those women who do suffer, whether minimally or to the extent that their experience controls their lives, this book will attempt to identify the symptoms of PAS and offer some methods for getting through each stage and, finally, to healing.

This book is not intended to be the only tool to achieve healing. On the contrary, it was written to help women recognize that PAS is a valid condition that results from abortion and that they are not the only ones who have experienced grief over something that society told them would be an easy solution to unplanned or unwanted pregnancy. Hopefully, the material we present will give them the confidence to seek more complete and thorough direction from professional therapists and counselors. This book is also intended to help relatives of women who have had abortions understand the emotional effects that abortion has on their loved one and enable them to identify PAS symptoms she may be experiencing. Additionally, the information is offered to volunteer crisis pregnancy counselors as well as professional counselors who want to learn more about PAS and the steps to healing.

Which women are likely to suffer from PAS?

While not all women who have abortions will be victims of PAS, all are subject to PAS because they have

---

[8]Rue, op. cit., p. 38.

experienced all four of the events that place people at a high risk of suffering from emotional problems: a sudden death, the death of a child, the sudden death of an infant, and survivor guilt.[9]

The women most likely to suffer from PAS will have experienced specific circumstances or possess certain characteristics:[10]

1. A maternal orientation.
2. Prior children.
3. Prior abortions.
4. Religious affiliation and conservatism.
5. No relationship support.
6. Have suffered forced abortions.
7. Second trimester abortions.
8. Genetic vs. elective abortions.
9. Pre-abortion experience of ambivalence.
10. Prior emotional problems.
11. Low in self-esteem.
12. Void of family of origin support.
13. Are of adolescent age rather than adult.

Of course, the more circumstances the woman has experienced or the more characteristics she has from the above list, the more likely she is to suffer from PAS and to a greater degree.

The woman who suffers heavily from PAS becomes severely depressed and loses pleasure in almost everything in life. She is likely to experience poor appetite, sleep disturbance, agitation of behavior, loss of pleasure

[9]Dr. E. Joanne Angelo, "Identifying Post Abortion Syndrome and Breaking Denial," presented at Healing Visions II, the Second National Conference on Post Abortion Counseling, University of Notre Dame (July 19, 1987).
[10]Dr. Vincent M. Rue, "Current Status and Trends in the Study of Post Abortion Syndrome," presented at Healing Visions II, the Second National Conference on Post Abortion Counseling, University of Notre Dame (July 19, 1987).

in usual activities, such as her sexual relationship(s), loss of energy, inappropriate guilt, a diminished ability to concentrate, and recurrent thoughts of suicide ("I just want to sleep" or "I wish to join my baby").[11]

A woman is at a greater risk of suffering from PAS when a new loss releases the problems of a previous, unresolved loss.[12] The woman must then acknowledge and cope with the grief she had denied in order to deal with the new loss. Even if the woman has been successful in her denial of previous losses, she is at greater risk of suffering emotional trauma when a new loss occurs.

Betty had a therapeutic abortion 20 years ago and then lost two other children at birth or shortly thereafter. She has not allowed herself to think about the abortion other than to tell herself that she had no choice in the matter because her doctor performed it without her real consent. She also has not allowed herself to mourn the deaths of the two other children to the extent that she has never visited their graves or had markers placed there. With all three deaths, she has denied her grief and sorrow. Recently, Betty's husband died quite unexpectedly and in her grief she is now remembering her previous losses. Betty is definitely at a high risk of suffering from PAS and needs to recognize that it is okay to grieve for the loss of her aborted child as well as her other two infants.

Special risks to adolescents

Every 2.1 minutes in the United States, a teenager conceives. Of the more than 1.1 million unintended teen pregnancies each year, half end in abortion or miscarriage.[13]

---

[11]Angelo, op. cit.

[12]Ibid.

[13]Dr. Vincent M. Rue, "Post Abortion Syndrome," presented at Healing Visions, the First National Conference on Post Abortion Counseling, University of Notre Dame (August 11, 1986), p. 49.

Teenagers who have abortions are at special risk to developing PAS because they are in a critical developmental period of their life. When we consider that emotional development continues into a person's 20's, then abortion by adolescents becomes a larger issue and we are now referring to the group of women upon which 50% of all abortions are performed: women who are 24 years old and younger.[14]

Not only are teens in a higher risk category for suffering from PAS, but their ability to successfully deliver healthy infants in future pregnancies is jeopardized. A pro-abortion professor of OB/GYN at the University of Newcastle-on-Tyne reported on his follow-up of 50 teenage mothers who had abortions performed by him. He reported that of their 53 subsequent pregnancies: 6 had another induced abortion, 19 had spontaneous miscarriages, 1 delivered a stillborn baby at 6 months, 6 babies died between birth and 2 years, and 21 babies survived.[15]

What percentage of teenagers opt for abortion? In a 1982 national survey of family growth, it was estimated that 18% of today's teens will have had an abortion by the age of 20, 41% by age 30, and 46% by age 45.[16] If these estimates are realized, the potential number of PAS sufferers is high.

Because adolescents will not deal emotionally with their abortion until five to ten years later, often when they are ready to start a family, their maturing process is delayed. The longer they delay dealing with the abortion,

---

[14]Dr. Wanda Franz, "Post Abortion Healing and the Adolescent," presented at Healing Visions II, the Second National Conference on Post Abortion Counseling, University of Notre Dame (July 20, 1987).

[15]Dr. & Mrs. J. C. Willke, *Abortion Questions & Answers* (Cincinnati, Ohio: Hayes Publishing Company, Inc., 1985), p. 109.

[16]Dr. Vincent M. Rue, "Current Status and Trends in the Study of Post Abortion Syndrome," presented at Healing Visions II, the Second National Conference on Post Abortion Counseling, University of Notre Dame (July 19, 1987).

the longer they will delay their adolescent stage.[17]

In addition, we need to recognize that teenagers are in the process of identifying who they are and are vulnerable to labels they give themselves. Teens having an abortion, who had believed that abortion is wrong and is done only by a bad person, may believe that they are totally evil and attempt to fulfill that image the rest of their lives.[18] They may feel they don't deserve the life that "good" people lead, so they will set themselves up to fail, whether it is at school, a job, or personal relationships.

Who is not likely to be affected by PAS?

Women who are less likely to be affected by PAS are those who rely heavily on rationalizing their actions. That is, they rely more on their thinking than on their feelings. Denial is part of their personality. They possess a wide range of feelings that are underdeveloped.[19] As long as they can maintain their system of rationalization, they will not likely be affected. But later losses, as mentioned earlier, may generate the need to grieve that will arouse the past abortion loss and force the woman to face the unresolved grief.

How a woman responds to abortion

Each woman's experience is unique to herself. Her reasons for having the abortion and her personal circumstances at the time of the abortion will vary. However, how a woman reacts to the experience can be categorized

---

[17]Franz, op. cit.
[18]Rev. Ken Metz, "Post Abortion Healing and the Adolescent," presented at Healing Visions II, the Second National Conference on Post Abortion Counseling, University of Notre Dame (July 20, 1987).
[19]Rue, op. cit.

into three distinct types: emotional, behavioral, and cognitive.[20]

The more common emotional responses include grief, guilt, anger, fear, and depression. A woman can experience several of these responses or all five.

Behavioral responses can be varied and include frequent crying, the inability to communicate with others concerning the pregnancy and abortion experience, flashbacks of the abortion experience, sexual inhibition, thoughts of suicide, and increased use of alcohol.

Cognitive responses are also varied. A common cognitive response after an abortion is the desire to learn more about pregnancy, fetal development, and abortion procedures. This can be stress reducing if it helps the woman integrate the abortion experience into her perceptual and belief system. It has been found that, initially, an increased knowledge of pregnancy and abortion enhances stress. The woman's new awareness of fetal development and the abortion method used for her own abortion can cause a great deal of guilt, anger, and depression, resulting in higher stress.[21]

Response to therapeutic abortions

A woman who has had a therapeutic abortion may believe that she has no reason to feel guilty or grieve because the choice for abortion was a medical decision, not a personal one. So she will deny any feelings of remorse and attempt to block her grief. She may not let herself think about the procedure, other than, "It had to be done. I had no choice."

---

[20]Dr. Anne Speckhard, "The Psycho-Social Aspects of Stress Following Abortion," Doctoral Thesis submitted to the University of Minnesota (May 1985), p. 109.
[21]Ibid., p. 110.

Later, if she feels guilt or sorrow, she will become confused about her emotions and worry that there is something mentally wrong. She may question, "Why do I feel this way if I had no choice in the matter and my doctor said I had to have the abortion?" Instead of dealing with her true feelings over her loss, she will condemn herself for being a weak person and not acting mature about a difficult situation.

Whether the abortion is elective or therapeutic, there is still the loss of a child, a death experience, that needs to be recognized by the woman.[22] In order for her to function in a healthy state of mind, she needs to deal with her emotional reactions to the abortion and allow herself to grieve the death of her child.

Defense mechanisms used by aborted women

Electing to have an abortion is a difficult decision, perhaps the most difficult decision a woman will ever make. Deep down, she knows it is wrong to take the life of the developing child within her. But circumstances prevent her from going through with the pregnancy, for one reason or another. So after perhaps weeks of struggling, she finally decides that she must abort her child, not realizing that she is creating an environment for even greater anguish and pain.

To cope with the emotional pain that accompanies abortion, the woman will develop a set of defense mechanisms to justify her decision. These defense mechanisms can be categorized into the following four types:[23]

1. *Rationalization*. These are the reasons a woman

---

[22]Rue, op. cit.

[23]Sr. Paula Vandegaer, "Current Status and Trends in the Development of Post Abortion Healing," presented at Healing Visions II, the Second National Conference on Post Abortion Counseling, University of Notre Dame (July 20, 1987).

gives for having an abortion that explain that what she is doing (or has done) is good. She might say, "I couldn't bring another unwanted child into the world" or "I can't give a child everything it needs in today's society" or "It was the best thing I could do under the circumstances." Rationalizations are very strong and important when supporting an action that might be perceived as bad. We don't want to choose evil; we must always choose the apparent good, so our rationalizations must support our actions as being good. Because rationalizations are very strong, it is difficult to talk a woman out of them. They are defenses against feelings she doesn't want to deal with.

When Kathy had her abortion in 1972, she rationalized that she had no other choice because she and her husband could not afford a baby at that time. They delayed the abortion until the 12th week of pregnancy because they didn't even have the money for an abortion. "I didn't believe abortion was wrong at the time, but then I didn't really understand it. It wasn't until the birth of our son four years later that I gave it any thought and then I had to deal with the guilt."

2. *Suppression*. This occurs when a woman erases any negative feelings about abortion from her mind. The feelings may occasionally emerge, but she will quickly put them out of her consciousness. To avoid these unwanted thoughts, the woman will not allow herself time to contemplate her personal feelings when they surface. If she is a Christian, she will avoid prayer time with God. She will keep herself busy with various activities so she doesn't have time to reflect or meditate. She might work two or more jobs or serve a cause as a volunteer, especially if the cause supports the woman's right to have an abortion.

Marta avoids conversations about abortion, keeping busy as an editor for a national magazine. No one at the office knows that she had an abortion as a college student twelve years ago. They see her as a caring person who works long hours at her job. When confronted with the abortion issue, she will simply maintain, "Science proves that there is no real life at conception; it's just a mass of tissue."

3. *Repression.* With repression, the woman is not aware of any negative feelings that she may have about the abortion. Much counseling must take place to bring back the repressed feelings in order for her to be healed emotionally. This can be a severe problem, because when we repress one feeling, we repress all feelings. Women repressing feelings about a past abortion will often act as if they are totally in charge of their lives.

Linda had an abortion during her first marriage. She doesn't believe there was anything wrong with having an abortion and has become a staunch supporter of women's rights. A career woman, she is very open about her desire to remain childless, noting that she is so happy when she sees a "wanted" baby born into a family. She has definite career goals and a lifestyle that leaves no room for children. Now remarried, she gives the impression that she is in control of her spouse and her future. While she maintains that she has happily chosen to remain childless, Linda speaks longingly about other people's young children. When she learned that her first husband had married a woman with children, she was very upset. "I always thought he didn't want children," she cried.

4. *Compensation.* This occurs when the woman becomes pregnant soon after her abortion to make up for the lost child. This subsequent pregnancy may be terminated through abortion or she may carry the baby to term. If she has another abortion, she may do so to reinforce her belief that abortion is a right and to maintain the sexual freedom she used with the first pregnancy. If she carries the baby

to term, the child often serves as a substitute for the aborted baby. The mother may give an excessive amount of attention to the child and try to become a "super mom." If the child has physical or behavioral problems, the mother may suffer excessive anxiety and feel as if she is being punished for her past abortion.

Ann aborted her first child because she wasn't married to the father and didn't want to pressure him into marriage with an unplanned pregnancy. Several months after the abortion, the couple married. Ann wanted to have a baby right away. Her pregnancy went well until the beginning of the eighth month, when Ann gave birth prematurely to a four-and-one-half pound girl. The baby suffered from respiratory complications and had to be hospitalized for four weeks. Ann blamed herself for the baby's problems and believes that she is being punished for her earlier abortion. She is very protective of her little girl and has told her husband that she doesn't want to have any more children.

Denial blocks healing

Through denial, the woman has blocked the natural grieving process for the death of her child, and often has denied her own responsibility for the decision to abort. This blockage of the healing process can lead to trauma that will become evident psychologically, physically, and spiritually.[24]

In addition to the woman's denial that a death has occurred, society has denied that abortion is a major death experience. According to Dr. Vincent Rue, noted clinical psychologist and authority on PAS, "The horror of a child's death is so overwhelming and frightening to us as

---

[24]*Post Abortion Syndrome . . . a reality*, brochure published by Victims of Choice, 2505 Wright Avenue, Pinole, CA 94565, p. 4.

a people that we must seek to protect ourselves under the mantle of denial and flee any feelings. We fear contamination somehow, if only in an emotional sense; we do not want to be touched by the instrument or illusion of death. . . . The agony that I have destroyed my unborn child's life is so heinous and threatening that the parent must suppress such a thought to survive, hiding this gnawing anguish in the deepest well of one's being. If it seeps into consciousness, it paralyzes and leaves one impotent to prevent, alter or deny it. By destroying unborn human life, parents are left unwhole. The dead child's space remains empty and the parents' emptiness becomes part of their very being, that is, if they allow themselves to feel."[25]

Denial is a strong defense mechanism used by the woman to suppress her feelings about the loss of her child. We will deal more in depth with this stage of PAS in Chapter Four. First, however, we will look at grief and how the grieving process for the aborted woman is unique.

---

[25]Dr. Vincent M. Rue, "Post Abortion Syndrome," presented at Healing Visions, the First National Conference on Post Abortion Counseling, University of Notre Dame (August 11, 1986), pp. 24–25.

CHAPTER THREE

GRIEF

Thirty-five-year-old Jane has undergone two abortions: one in 1972 and another three years later. Both times, she had a very casual relationship with the fathers of the aborted babies, so she arranged to have the abortions without their knowledge. She didn't share her experiences with any friends and didn't talk about the abortions.

"I couldn't tell anyone about the abortions," Jane said. "I felt very low and that I was causing everyone problems. The only people who knew about my first abortion were my parents and a younger brother."

After her first abortion, Jane felt very confused and empty inside. She attended many parties where she drank large quantities of alcohol, trying to forget who she was. She longed to be accepted and wanted someone to make her happy, which is how she ended up getting pregnant again.

"I couldn't tell anyone about the second pregnancy because that proved I was no good. I figured the only way out was abortion. And it was so easy because there was a clinic in town. I called them, they did a pregnancy test and scheduled me for an abortion. No one talked to me about alternatives or gave me any information about the abortion procedure. I was very scared."

When she arranged for her second abortion, Jane didn't intend to tell anyone but changed her mind after she arrived at the clinic. She decided to call her mother to let her know her plans in case something went wrong.

At the clinic, she volunteered to be the first of ten women to have her abortion. "I wanted to get it over with and get out of there. The doctor started up a motor that was really loud. The pain was very intense and I felt as if my insides were being torn out. No one referred to my pain or what I might be feeling. It was like I was just a small part of their day's work; it was just a business procedure."

After the abortion, a woman led Jane to another room to rest. She felt very weak. The woman told her she could get dressed and go home when she was ready. The woman handed her a piece of paper with instructions of things to do and not do for the next week. "Basically, she just said to take care of myself the best you know how," Jane said. "There was no checkup scheduled or calls to see how I was getting along."

As Jane walked down the stairs, she saw her mother sitting in the waiting room. Her obvious concern touched Jane's heart, but she felt too ashamed to confide in her and tell her how much she hurt inside. "She wanted to comfort me, but I didn't want to talk to her about it. I felt worthless."

Even though Jane refused to talk about her two abortions with friends or counselors, they had an immediate effect on her emotional life.

The reality of what she had done began to bother Jane. Pangs of guilt gradually developed into a constant self-talk of being a terrible person and totally worthless. Life lost all meaning. Jane said, "I remember thinking, 'What kind of person would kill her own children? I must be a really terrible woman and I don't deserve to live.' "

Church had been a part of Jane's life as a child. During her years after high school she had grown away from it. As memories of her second abortion began to plague her every waking thought, Jane sought solace in church services. "But instead of being comforted, I felt worse. I couldn't sit through an entire service without crying. I still wasn't sharing my experiences with anyone, and I couldn't understand why I seemed to have no control over my thoughts or actions. It got to the point where I was a physical mess. I couldn't sleep at night and I didn't take care of myself. I was becoming anorexic and didn't care about my appearance or health. I was thinking so much about my abortions and the fact that I had killed two human beings; the accusing thoughts were always there. I had no self-worth. I was very, very fearful of myself, and didn't want to be alone, for fear of what I might do to punish myself."

Although Jane didn't realize it, she was experiencing various aspects of grief: mourning the loss of her dead children and feeling tremendous guilt, so much guilt to the extent that it made her physically ill and so emotionally unstable that she became suicidal. Even though she recognized the reality of her abortions, she didn't understand that the emotional stress she suffered was caused by her guilt over the abortions and her inability to knowingly grieve for the loss of her two children.

What is grief?

Grief is a process of emotional suffering, usually caused by the loss of someone or something very special to us. Distress, affliction, sorrow, painful regret, bereavement, remorse, and despair are all descriptions of grief.[1] Grief can be very intense and last for years or it can appear momentarily in our lives, such as when we watch a sad ending to a movie.

In most cases, we know we are grieving because an event has occurred, such as the death of a parent or other loved one, that society has told us we are expected to grieve. For some people, grief is a devastating experience that totally destroys a normal pattern of living. They might lie in bed all day, sit listlessly in a chair or cry for no apparent reason. For others, grief is short-lived and affects their daily living pattern for only a little while.

But what happens when we grieve about something that society does not expect us to grieve about? Are we even aware that we are grieving? And how do we resolve this apparent conflict?

Such grieving occurs after an abortion. That's really what Post Abortion Syndrome (PAS) is all about: the stress that a woman may suffer after she's had an abortion. The stress results when she feels the need to grieve but she doesn't recognize this need or allow it to occur.

Who grieves?

Is grief reserved only for a few select women who are more emotional or sensitive about babies? Is this a rare occurrence among women who abort?

In her 1985 thesis entitled "Psycho-Social Aspects of Stress Following Abortion,"[2] Dr. Anne Speckhard found that 100% of the women in her survey who aborted had experienced feelings of grief, sadness, regret or loss. Com-

---

[1] Webster's Third New International Dictionary (Springfield, Mass.: G. & C. Merriam Company, 1976), pp. 998–999.

[2] Dr. Anne Speckhard, "The Psycho-Social Aspects of Stress Following Abortion," Doctoral Thesis submitted to the University of Minnesota (May, 1985), pp. 92–93, 106.

mon reactions following their abortions were frequent crying (81%) and thoughts of suicide (65%). In her study group, 81% of the women were preoccupied with the aborted child and 73% experienced flashbacks of the abortion.

Not all women who grieve will suffer from PAS. On the contrary, women who allow themselves to grieve and understand their need to grieve are not likely to experience PAS. However, many women won't allow themselves to grieve over their aborted child. In order for them to agree to the abortion, they have convinced themselves that they aren't aborting a child, only a potential life. Therefore, there is nothing to grieve about. In addition, their doctor, and other people who may know about the abortion, will very likely have told them that abortion is merely a medical procedure to correct a mistake. So any symptoms of grief that arise must be ignored by the woman if she is to continue believing she did the right thing by choosing abortion.

How can a woman grieve for an unwanted child?

"Do you want this pregnancy?" is a question routinely asked by a woman's doctor. We live in an age when our desire to have a baby determines whether the fetus will be allowed to grow and develop and, eventually, be born. "Wantedness" by the mother for her child appears to be the sole criteria for birth.

According to Dr. Jean Garton in her book *Who Broke the Baby?*, wantedness of the child does not tell us anything about the child but about the mother. "When I say, 'You are 'wanted' or 'unwanted,' " whom am I describing? Not you! Rather, I would be telling you something about myself, for 'wantedness' measures the emotions and the feelings of the 'want-er.' . . . The unwanted child is the victim not of his own shortcomings but of those in a society attempting to solve its social, economic and personal problems by the sacrificial offering of its children."[3]

Dr. Garton explains that often the condition of pregnancy is unwanted, not the baby. "Medical studies indicate that for many women, including those whose pregnancies are planned, the condition of pregnancy with its many hormonal and physical changes initially may be unwanted. Yet given the passage of time and supportive counseling, the child of the pregnancy becomes very wanted."[4]

So, when the woman says she doesn't want her baby, she could be saying she doesn't want this pregnancy, this inconvenience, this added financial burden, this infringement on her freedom, this commitment for the next 18 years or so. She may want the baby; she doesn't want the changes in her lifestyle that a baby requires.

Counselor Terry Selby reports that 25% of his therapy patients who have had abortions and who relive the abortion experience in therapy will begin to shake and cry out, aware that they are reliving the death agony of their child which they had sensed even as the abortion was taking place.[5] They are, in fact, grieving for their baby who is being killed, a baby they thought they didn't want.

Selby's findings are supported by healing ministry teachers and authors Dennis and Matthew Linn, S.J. and Sheila Fabricant, M. Div. "Our experience in inner-healing prayer confirms that women who choose to abort a child grieve for their babies. We have often prayed with

---

[3]Dr. Jean Garton, *Who Broke the Baby?* (Minneapolis, Minn.: Bethany House Publishers, 1979), p. 30.

[4]Ibid., p. 31.

[5]Dennis and Matthew Linn, S.J., and Sheila Fabricant, M. Div., "Healing Relationships with Miscarried, Aborted, and Stillborn Babies," *Journal of Christian Healing* (Vol. 7, No. 2), p. 35.

women who, many years after an abortion, still struggled with unresolved grief."[6]

So, even though she may deny wanting a child, the woman who aborts will grieve for the child's loss, whether knowingly or unknowingly.

It's important to understand that not all aborted children are "unwanted." Their mothers really do want them, but they are overwhelmed by their current situation and don't see how they can handle having a baby at this point in their lives. They may be greatly influenced by friends, counselors, and their doctor to have the abortion, when, deep inside, they want someone to show them how it will all work out and they can have their baby. These women especially need to knowingly grieve for their loss and should seek the help of Christian counselors.

Is all grief alike?

Our society became educated about the grieving process in Elisabeth Kubler-Ross's book *On Death and Dying*. She taught us that there are five stages a person goes through when they are confronted with death through a terminal illness. She identified these stages as denial and isolation, anger, bargaining, depression, and acceptance.[7] Not surprisingly, these are almost identical to the stages that a person goes through when they grieve after an abortion.

According tc Dr. Anne Speckhard, the five stages to the grieving process for a woman who has had an abortion are denial, bargaining, anger, depression, and acceptance.[8] A woman may experience these stages in any or-

---

[6]Ibid., p. 35.

[7]Elisabeth Kubler-Ross, *On Death and Dying* (New York: Macmillan Company, 1969), pp. 34, 44, 72, 75, 99.

[8]Dr. Anne Speckhard, "Diagnosis and Treatment of Post Abortion Syndrome," clinical skills training workshop held in Cedar Rapids, Iowa (June 18, 1987).

der, but denial almost always occurs first.

Even though this woman's grief can be broken down into stages similar to grief experienced by a dying person and others who are grieving for loved ones, there are special qualities to her grief. Boston psychiatrist Dr. Joanne Angelo has found in her counseling experience specific differences in the grief of a woman who has aborted. "Grief after an abortion is complex, difficult, and prolonged. The person you are grieving for has been the victim of a violent, sudden death. Typically, the mother is alone and does not deal with the loss until several years after it has occurred. There is no wake or funeral and no visual memory of the baby. Her only memory is the frightening recall of the abortion procedure, which can be brought on by the whir of the vacuum or a visit to the dentist."[9]

In addition, Dr. Angelo said, the mother experiences mood swings with the hormonal changes her body undergoes, from the state of not being pregnant to being pregnant to not being pregnant again. She also feels a deep sense of guilt and repeatedly will remind herself (as Jane did), "I am the murderer of a child." This sense of guilt will separate her from her family and from God. She feels unlovable and may develop suicidal thoughts.[10]

In her book *Helping People Through Grief*, Delores Kuenning supports the thought that grief suffered as the result of an abortion is unlike any other loss and identifies nine problems related to a woman's mourning the loss of an aborted baby:[11]

---

[9]Dr. E. Joanne Angelo, "The Healing Process," presented at Healing Visions, the First National Conference on Post Abortion Counseling, University of Notre Dame (August 12, 1986).

[10]Ibid., audio cassette available through the National Youth Pro-Life Coalition, Jackson Avenue, Hastings-on-Hudson, NY 10706.

[11]Delores A. Kuenning, *Helping People Through Grief* (Minneapolis, Minn.: Bethany House Publishers, 1987), pp. 179–181.

1. There is no external evidence that a baby ever existed, so there is no proof that she was even pregnant. Her baby lives only in her mind and heart.

2. There is no formal leave-taking or ritual, such as a funeral, for the mother where friends and loved ones can acknowledge her loss and share her grief.

3. The woman has no support system because usually few people are told about the abortion.

4. Although legal, abortion is still socially unacceptable, so no one gives her permission to grieve openly. She must suffer in secret.

5. The woman carries the guilt of ending her baby's life. Many women can't seem to forgive themselves, and live in pain and isolation.

6. If she shares what she did with a loved one, she may experience rejection, disapproval, anger, humiliation, and harsh judgment. This reaction to her deed may prove to be devastating, especially when she is already feeling guilty and alone.

7. Few professional counselors have been trained to take these women through the steps necessary for healing and reconciliation with God.

8. Abortion advocates provide no classes or education to prepare the woman for the tremendous sense of loss they will feel after abortion.

9. The grief cycle and timing is different than other types of losses. A woman may remain in a stage of denial for years and postpone the grieving process. Usually, grief over an abortion loss is most intense in the initial stages.

Abortion grief is unique, and many women can be helped to acknowledge and unblock this grieving process through Christian counseling. By recognizing their need to grieve and allowing it to occur, women who aborted are taking steps to prevent PAS from controlling their lives.

How long will the woman who aborted grieve?

How long the woman who aborted grieves depends on her individual experience and her personal strengths and resources. Usually, the more unstable her family background, the more traumatic her abortion experience will be.[12] When her resources are inadequate or continually overwhelmed by intense psychic overload, traumatization follows.[13]

In most cases, the woman who aborted has created and adopted a set of emotional and psychological defenses that have not allowed her to face the reality of her abortion. She begins rationalizing her decision the moment she considers abortion, continues as she develops reasons to abort her child, and is complete when the procedure is finished. This system of rationalizing is the basis for later emotional, psychological, and relational problems.[14] The woman also utilizes a thinking system that includes facts, real experience, personal beliefs, and values. This system carries the information that is contrary to her decision to abort and must be acknowledged before the guilt and shame can be resolved. As the actual traumatic experience of the woman becomes more real to her, she is better able to regain control of her thinking, feelings, and actions. She begins to accept the thoughts and feelings that she has kept private or suppressed. As she is able to acknowledge to herself and to others the traumatic experience of the abortion and its emotional effects, the better she feels and is able to cope.

How long she grieves depends on how long she ra-

---

[12]Dr. Vincent Rue, "Post Abortion Syndrome," presented at Healing Visions, the First National Conference on Post Abortion Counseling, University of Notre Dame (August 11, 1986), p. 33.
[13]Ibid., pp. 34 and 36.
[14]Terry L. Selby, "Post Abortion Trauma," unpublished paper, copyright 1984, p. 12. Copy may be obtained by contacting Counseling Associates of Bemidji, Inc., P.O. Box 577, Bemidji, MN 56601.

tionalizes her abortion before she deals with her real feelings about the whole experience.[15]

How to identify unresolved grief

When grief is allowed to run its normal course, it is a healing process. That is, we allow ourselves to grieve, we acknowledge that we are grieving, and we find peace within ourselves. But there is a difference between resolved grief and unresolved grief. Unresolved grief is more common among women who are in the denial stage and not dealing with their symptoms of grief. Grief cannot be avoided; it must be accepted and dealt with before it can be resolved.

In Jane's case, she did not acknowledge the feelings she experienced as the result of her abortions. She wouldn't talk to anyone about what she had been through and attempted to go on living as if nothing had happened. But the memories crept into her thinking and she would cry for no apparent reason; she felt guilty but didn't understand why because abortion was legal and so easy to arrange. "I told myself there was no reason for being upset," Jane said.

Every woman grieves in her own way as the result of her abortion experience, just as people in general react differently to grief experiences. Colin Parkes, a senior research psychiatrist at the Tavistoch Institute of Human Relations in London, has identified seven types of grief reactions:[16]

1. *A process of realization.* With abortion, this would occur when the woman moves from denying that abortion is a death experience or that she has suffered a loss to

---

[15]Ibid., p. 13.
[16]Joan Pincus, "Grief in Adoption and Abortion," *Heartbeat* (Spring 1984), p. 13.

accepting that a life has been taken.

2. *An alarm reaction.* The woman who aborted begins to experience anxiety, restlessness, and other symptoms that indicate that she feels uncomfortable with her decision to abort.

3. *An urge to search for and to find the lost person in some form.* The woman who chose abortion may attempt to seek her lost child by again becoming pregnant. Or, she may search for pictures of an aborted fetus at the age her baby was at the time of the abortion. She will devour information on fetal development in medical books and spend much time examining plastic fetal models. She wants to know what her baby looked like so she can attach her grief to a specific image.

4. *Anger and guilt.* The woman will often feel anger toward the people who urged premature acceptance of grief. These are the friends who told her, "Sure, you feel bad now. But you'll get over it. It's really no big thing." Or she might be angry with her doctor who said, "I'm just going to remove a mass of tissue. You'll feel little pain and be back to normal in a day or two." On the contrary, she felt great pain and her life has not gotten back to normal.

5. *Feelings of internal loss of self.* The woman who aborted will feel as if she doesn't know herself, this person who could agree to an abortion. She will also feel empty inside.

6. *Identification phenomena.* This occurs when the woman adopts traits and mannerisms of the lost child. She may become childlike and unable to cope with her daily activities. She will want someone to take care of her.

7. *Pathological variants of grief.* Instead of experiencing the normal grief reactions, the woman who aborts will suffer from unwholesome thinking. For example, she may hate herself so much that she will contemplate suicide

and perhaps even attempt to take her own life.

According to Parkes, unresolved grief occurs somewhere between the fourth and fifth types of reactions, when the person becomes encompassed by his or her grief.[17]

If you've had an abortion

You suspect that you are experiencing unresolved abortion grief. These conditions may characterize you: Your life is consumed by feelings of worthlessness and self-reproach. You are angry at the people who told you abortion would be a quick solution to your problem. You think you have put your experience behind you, but then you cry for no reason about the same time every month. How can you know if you have resolved your grief?

Your answers to the following questions may reveal if you have resolved your abortion grief:

- Have I returned to my previous, pre-abortion level of functioning?
- Have I put away my defenses of denial?
- Have I experienced my child as having been real and mourned the loss appropriately?
- Can I imagine my baby at peace with God?
- Do I believe that God can forgive me?
- Have I asked God to forgive me?
- Have I accepted His forgiveness?
- Have I forgiven myself?
- Have I found meaning in this tragedy?

If you answer no to any of these questions, then you probably are suffering from unresolved grief over your abortion experience.

---

[17]Ibid., p. 13.

The rest of this book can help you, with God's help, to work through your grief and seek additional counseling resources. The following chapters will discuss each step in the grieving process and identify the techniques for working through each stage. Keep in mind that every woman does not progress through each step in the same order. So if you are depressed but haven't experienced anger, then first read the chapter on depression and fear. If you're unsure what stage you are in, then read the chapters in order. As you read, you will identify where you are in your grieving process so you can begin your healing.

CHAPTER FOUR

DENIAL

I didn't realize that having an abortion would kill my baby. I thought that I had to have it done because my doctor told me I would die if I gave birth."

Thirteen years after the abortion of her eight-week-old fetus, Jill is beginning to allow herself to grieve and to understand her need to grieve. She has denied the death of her baby until now because she didn't understand the abortion process or fetal development.

At the time of her abortion, Jill and her two young sons from her first marriage lived with her boyfriend. He didn't want to marry Jill or raise the child she carried—his child. He told her she had to get rid of "it" or lose him. At the same time, Jill's doctor strongly recommended an abortion because her recent stomach surgery had left her muscles weak and unable to support a pregnancy. He told Jill, "A baby would kill you." Her doctor wouldn't perform the abortion, but referred her to a clinic.

Although abortion had recently become legal throughout the United States. Jill was confused about what getting an abortion really meant. "I knew I was pregnant, but I really didn't understand that I was carrying a baby. I didn't know anything about the development of the baby and I didn't ask any questions. I only heard the doctor say I had to have an abortion or I would die."

Afraid of losing her boyfriend and endangering her own life, Jill contacted the abortionist and made an appointment for the next week. Doubts about what she planned to do crept into her mind, but she shut them out, reminding herself that she had no choice in the matter.

Miles from home, Jill felt alone in the cold, sterile clinic with an unfriendly doctor who seemed too busy to talk to her and who never used the word "abortion." Jill did not receive counseling or an explanation of what would happen to her. Afraid to ask, she did not want to find out details that might upset her. The doctor performed the procedure swiftly and without incident. The bleeding that followed concerned Jill. They told her it would stop after a few days and she should take it easy.

Jill returned home to discover that her problems were only beginning. "I was an emotional and physical wreck. I cried a lot and was very depressed. Before I had been outgoing but afterward I reacted to the slightest thing. I couldn't stand babies or hold down my job." She lost all desire to get up in the morning. She would sit for hours, staring at nothing. She managed to care for her sons' basic needs, but everything she did for them became an effort. She began to resent them.

Jill's boyfriend didn't offer any support. He had hinted that if she had the abortion, they would get married, and he would plant a tree in remembrance of the baby they could have had together. But his words proved to be lies, spoken only to convince Jill that abortion was her one and only option. Within one month, their relationship had totally fallen apart, and Jill moved out of their apartment and back with her parents, who had no knowledge of her abortion.

Jill's life slowly began to fall apart. She felt tormented, out of control, and she didn't understand why. She began drinking heavily and her need to smoke pot increased. Only when she was high could Jill escape the anxiety that tormented her every waking hour. Ultimately she suffered a nervous breakdown and was hospitalized for six months.

While she suffered emotionally, Jill also battled the physical effects of her abortion. "I bled heavily because my uterus had been perforated during the abortion. It also caused my female organs to drop, as well as my liver and kidneys. I would bleed for two weeks every time I had a period, which resulted in a constant infection. My family doctor, the one who had originally recommended the abortion, wouldn't treat me. I was too ashamed to go to another doctor because I would have to tell him about the abortion. So I lived with the bleeding and pain for 12 years."

Jill buried the memory of her abortion and never talked about it with anyone. But the crying and depression continued.

Despite her inner turmoil, Jill lived what appeared to be a happy life. She fell in love with a man who married her and wanted to care for her and her two sons. But she didn't tell her husband about her abortion and constantly struggled with feelings of self-hatred. Even the birth of a son, nine years after her abortion, did not erase the torment Jill combatted daily. She couldn't understand why she verbally and physically abused her husband and children, who were equally confused by her anger.

Even as a Christian, Jill did not feel she could go to God with her emotional problems. In her mind, God, as the authority figure, would condemn her for what she had done.

One day Jill met a woman her own age and they soon

became good friends. Her new friend, active in the area right-to-life organization, told Jill about the group's activities and how abortion can devastate women's lives. She explained that many women experience guilt and anger because they have lost a child but don't realize the need to grieve over their loss. Their denial causes much emotional pain and anxiety.

Jill listened to her friend describe the effects abortion has on a woman and thought, "She's describing me!" Then the word abortion reached down into Jill's past and brought back the memory of her own experience. Suddenly, it all made sense—the guilt, the torment, the anger. Relief flooded her. She wasn't losing her mind! The terrible experiences of the last 12 years were all reactions to her abortion.

Once Jill acknowledged her abortion, she could deal with what she had done and her responsibility for it. After years of denying the abortion by not talking about it with anyone or even allowing herself to dwell on it, Jill was now ready to work through her feelings. Jill identified the emotional effects of abortion in her life and saw the need to grieve for her dead baby. She also realized that her anger was directed at the people who influenced her abortion decision—the doctor, her boyfriend, and herself. Through prayer, Jill found forgiveness, both for the people who told her she had to have the abortion, and for herself.

What is denied?

Post Abortion Syndrome encompasses the mourning, guilt, pain and grief that has been denied. The longer a woman denies her abortion and her responsibility for it, the more intense her reactions to the abortion.[1] The basis

---

[1] Dr. Vincent Rue, "Post Abortion Syndrome," presented at Healing Visions, the First National Conference on Post Abortion Counseling, University of Notre Dame (August 11, 1986), p. 32.

of her denial is the fact that abortion took the life of her child and she allowed it to happen.

When Jill acknowledged that her abortion caused her emotional problems, she confronted what she had denied for 12 years—the loss of her child. Confronting the death of a child is the first step to healing when coping with Post Abortion Syndrome.

Why deny death?

In his paper "Post Abortion Syndrome," psychologist Dr. Vincent Rue relates that the relationship between parent and child is like no other in its uniqueness and complexity. By killing the unborn child, abortion attempts to end the bonding process that begins when a woman first learns she is pregnant. "Abortion creates an immediate void in the parent characterized by ambivalence, emptiness and confusion. As the fetal child dies, so also does a part of the parent, male or female, married or not, minor or adult. Abortion is not just 'pregnancy termination' or 'cellular disposal.' It is a personal and relational amputation. Parents are parents forever, even of a dead child."[2]

For Jill, her abortion was a necessary procedure to prevent health problems for herself. She believed that if she continued the pregnancy, she would lose the baby anyway, because her body could not carry the pregnancy to term. In order to allow the abortion to occur, she told herself that she terminated a pregnancy, never admitting a life had been taken. As a result, she felt confused and empty inside. She didn't understand her frequent crying and depression. She didn't realize that her feelings were the result of the denial that a death had occurred.

The woman uses denial, then, to protect herself from

----

[2]Ibid., p. 24.

experiencing abortion death, which brings with it anxiety, guilt, and, often, anger.

Father Michael Mannion, college campus minister and author of *Abortion & Healing, A Cry to Be Whole*, says that women deny death in abortion so they can deny that what they have done is a wrong act separating themselves from God, a sin. "The aborted woman feels far from God because she has denied that abortion is a sin. She will try to rationalize her actions but will realize, deep inside, that no degree of rationalization will convince God of her innocence."[3]

So whether she is a Christian woman or someone who doesn't profess a faith but believes in a supreme being, the woman who aborts employs denial, first, to negate the death of a human child and, second, to disavow the fact that the intentional death goes against God's will.

Types of denial

According to Dr. Rue, there are various types and degrees of denial, from mild to severe.[4]

Occluded. In this type of denial, the woman has no conscious awareness of the pain or loss. She might say, "I never had an abortion." Basically, she is hiding all emotions and feelings that the abortion may have triggered. She buries them deep in her subconscious where she won't ever have to deal with them.

Deb used this type of denial for three of her four abortions. She didn't allow herself to think about the abortions or feel anything afterward. Drugs and alcohol helped her repress any thoughts she might have had. During her

---

[3]Father Michael T. Mannion, S.T.L., M.A., "Post Abortion Reconciliation," presented at Healing Visions, the First National Conference on Post Abortion Counseling, University of Notre Dame (August 13, 1986), taped lecture.
[4]Rue, op. cit., pp. 25–27.

fourth abortion when the doctor said to her, "How many more of these do you think you can have?" Deb finally considered the physical and emotional effects of abortion. Then feelings of guilt and anxiety began to surface.

Phantom Pregnancy. With this type of denial, the woman believes she is still pregnant and acts as if she is pregnant. She may wear maternity clothes and even show physical signs of pregnancy, such as weight gain.

Fourteen weeks into her pregnancy, Denise had begun to feel fetal movements and had told several people about her pregnancy. Her parents threatened to throw her out of the house if she didn't have an abortion. Unmarried and unemployed, Denise said the pressure from her parents convinced her to have the abortion. After the procedure, Denise continued to believe that she was pregnant and began wearing maternity clothes. She ate more at mealtime, explaining that she now ate "for two." Despite her parents' insistence that she was not pregnant, Denise talked, walked and lived as if she were. Denise could not accept the fact of her abortion and baby's death until after she received professional counseling.

Obliteration. This occurs when the aborted woman attempts to erase all memory of both the pregnancy and the abortion. She lives as if they never occurred. She may experience pain and depression but she won't relate them to her abortion. This was the type of denial employed by Jill.

Periodic Denial. In this denial, the woman blocks the abortion trauma whenever she finds herself in a situation where she is reminded of her abortion. She does not grieve because, whenever feelings of remorse surface, she denies their existence. She won't allow herself to feel any emotions and begins to take on a "cold" attitude toward people and events that used to make her feel sad or cry.

Mona gets angry when she is reminded of her abortion

and realizes her anger is directed against her husband. She won't allow herself to grieve over their aborted child, however, and admits that she feels hardened against the sad things in life: hurting children, dying people, tragedies.

Compensatory Denial. This creates a distraction and a new emotional investment. A woman exhibits this type of denial by rushing into another activity as an outlet for her accumulated anxiety. These activities might include workaholism, a substitutional pregnancy or atonement child, sexual hyperactivity, or indulgence in chemical dependency.

Such was the case with Nancyjo. After her saline abortion, Nancyjo became sexually active, leaving her children with her mother while she visited local bars in search of men. Soon she used drugs and alcohol in her attempt to forget the abortion and the perfectly formed face that had stared up at her from the hospital basin. Gradually, she turned her anger inward and lost all self-esteem. She took risks, unconcerned about her health or safety. Only after she was nearly killed in a motorcycle accident did Nancyjo come to grips with her lifestyle, and subsequently, her abortion.

Segmented Denial. The most commonly employed following abortion, segmented denial enables the woman to recognize the abortion and/or loss of the fetal child, but protects herself against painful feelings associated with the abortion. If she uses this type of denial, the woman is unable to appropriately feel and/or mourn the loss created by the abortion.

Robin said that after her abortion she wanted to forget the whole thing. She moved halfway across the country in her attempt to put her past behind her. She left her parents who had not supported her abortion decision and the father of her aborted baby who had wanted to marry her. She planned to start over, with no reminders of her abortion or her life before the abortion.

Purposive Denial. With this form of denial, the woman rejects her feelings of grief when talking to other people for fear of embarrassment or shame, but admits to herself the wrongfulness of her actions. By carrying this private burden that becomes heavier with age, she becomes depressed, detached, disengaged, impersonal and unavailable to others.

At first, Kathy felt guilty for having aborted her baby, but when she sought counseling from a social service agency and her own pastor, they told her she had no reason to feel guilty. "I felt something must be wrong with me for having these feelings," Kathy said, so she didn't talk about them to anyone after that; she kept them inside. The guilt continued to torture Kathy. "I thought I was strong enough to cope with anything and as life went on for me, I kept pushing thoughts and guilt down to the empty pit within me."[5]

Type of denial determines stress level

In a recent study, psychologists Larry Cohen, M.A., and Susan Roth, Ph.D., evaluated the coping styles of 55 women who had aborted. As a group, the average distress level (marked by anxiety, depression, and denial) was fairly high. But Cohen and Roth found that when divided into groups, the women they termed "avoiders" experienced more distress than "approachers." And "approachers" decreased in distress over time while "avoiders" did not.[6]

---

[5]Kathy Bucklew, *My Private Story*, brochure published by Lutherans For Life, St. Paul, MN.

[6]Larry Cohen, M.A., and Susan Roth, Ph.D., "Coping with Abortion," *Journal of Human Stress* (Fall 1984), pp. 140–145.

In this study, avoiders were characterized by trying not to talk about the abortion, staying away from reminders of their experience, and avoiding becoming upset when they were reminded of the abortion. Approachers would talk about their experience, think of ways to prevent it from happening again, and try to deal with their resulting feelings.[7]

If you've had an abortion

Perhaps you're saying to yourself, "I had an abortion and haven't suffered any negative effects." According to Canadian clinician Ian Kent, M.D., the very absence of effect is really an emotional numbness, a significant negative effect in itself. Dr. Kent believes that the hurt of abortion is so deep that it is repressed and will rarely be revealed outside a deep trust relationship.[8]

Have you experienced some of the symptoms described in this book? Do you see yourself at one point or another in this stage we call denial? Then ask yourself this question: Am I ready to move on, to deal with the emotions I've been harboring, whether it has been for two weeks or 20 years?

If you answered yes, then here's what you can do.

According to psychologist Dr. William Backus, you must first recognize and free yourself from untruths that you have been carrying with you since before your abortion. The untruths are misbeliefs about the circumstances surrounding your abortion, the reasons behind your actions, and the effect that carrying the pregnancy to term would have had on your life. These are the answers you

[7]Ibid., pp. 140–145.
[8]Dennis and Matthew Linn, S.J., and Sheila Fabricant, M. Div., "Healing Relationships with Miscarried, Aborted, and Stillborn Babies," *Journal of Christian Healing* (Vol. 7, No. 2), p. 35.

gave yourself whenever doubts or guilt crept into your mind and accused you of making the wrong decision. These untruths enabled you to rationalize your decision and go through with the abortion.[9]

You need to especially target your misbeliefs about (1) how you have devalued yourself, (2) how you have devalued your daily life, and (3) how you have devalued your future. The following are some common misbeliefs of women who have had abortions, and why they are wrong:[10]

- I'm no good because of what I've done. (Your abortion decision was bad, but you are a good person.)
- I'm a failure at life. (One mistake, no matter what it is, does not make you a failure. You can admit your mistake, ask for God's forgiveness, and learn from your experience.)
- I don't deserve any happiness. (All people are sinners and none of us "deserves" happiness. It is only through the grace of God that our slate can be wiped clean and we can claim the victory over sin that Jesus has won for us.)
- I must always pay for what I've done. (As hard as you might try, you can never pay for your abortion. Christ has done that for you. All you need do is believe that He is your Savior and that He offers to you the gift of forgiveness. In return, you can show your gratitude by using your experience as a witness of His love. Tell others what Christ's love means to you and what effect it has had on your life.)

---

[9]William Backus, Ph.D., *Telling the Truth to Troubled People*, Fourth National Lutherans For Life Convention, November 2, 1985, Minneapolis, MN, workshop notes.
[10]Ibid.

- I will never get over it; I'm stuck with the consequences for the rest of my life. (This is your choice. As a forgiven Christian, you are set free from your bondage of sin, including your abortion, and can live a new life as a forgiven child of God.)
- It was only a fetus, I must not grieve. (You aborted a real person, not just a fetus. That person was your child and will no longer be a part of your life on earth. You have lost a precious gift and you have every right to grieve.)
- I shouldn't have to live with any remorse. (Remorse, by itself, is not productive. But if you allow it to lead you to repentance and to seek God's forgiveness, then it is a good thing.)
- I have to be perfect and I can't conceive of making a mistake. (None of us is perfect; all are sinners in God's eyes. We all make mistakes, but through God's grace, we can all be forgiven.)
- What others think is vitally important. (The most important thing is what God thinks about your life. Does it please Him or do you need to make some changes?)

According to Terry Selby, M.S.W., who counsels women at the nation's only in-patient treatment center for Post Abortion Syndrome, confronting denial (telling oneself the truth) is a two-step process:[11]

1. Recognize the emotional pain and grief you have experienced since your abortion. A recurring pain may occur whenever you see a new mother with a tiny infant or a child who is the age yours would have been, if he or

---

[11]Terry L. Selby, M.S.W., "Post Abortion Trauma," unpublished paper, copyright 1984 by Terry Selby, Counseling Associates, P.O. Box 577, Bemidji, MN, p. 4.

she had been allowed to live. Maybe you avoid pictures of children or cute television commercials depicting toddlers' mischievous actions. Or, early in the morning or late at night, you are tormented by a tiny voice calling to you.

Go over the details of your abortion, as you may have done many times before, but this time, react to what is happening. Don't cover up your feelings. Acknowledge the fear you felt when the doctor began dilating your cervix to a size that would accommodate the suction machine. Remember your racing heart and your cold sweaty hands and your shaking knees. Cry when you feel your baby being sucked from your womb. Feel the anguish and heartache.

2. Acknowledge that abortion is not just a procedure but it is the act of ending a tiny life. Then accept your responsibility for the abortion and death of your child. The "fetus" was in fact your child and your child is now dead. Say, "My baby is dead," and, "I was responsible for the death."

One method for recognizing that it was indeed your baby that was killed is to first bring back all the memories of the past. Talk about the facts and feelings that led to the abortion decision. Describe the abortion event itself. If you feel comfortable, write down on paper what happened. This way, you can be sure to include all the details and refer back to what happened, if you choose, at a later time. Also, the physical action of writing down your experience will prove to be therapeutic. Start big and move to detail. For example, list the name of the town where the abortion was performed, then move on to the part of the city, the name of the clinic or hospital, the time of day, the kind of day (weatherwise), and how you got to the abortion facility. Go back through your story again and again, each time adding more detail. You will probably experience some physical effects as your abortion becomes very real to you once again. Your body may shake and your teeth may chatter. You are experiencing fear, which we will discuss in Chapter Six.[12]

Once you've broken through your denial that a death occurred, you must give life to your baby. You can do this mentally by imagining what your baby would have looked like at birth. Picture his or her color of eyes and hair. (This is not to be confused with "New Age" visualization techniques.) Would he have your smile or she her father's eyes? Decide what sex your baby is and choose a name. This will give you a mental image of what your baby looks like to replace the incomplete or bloody memory you may have. Spend a little time getting to know your baby, to do some of the things that you had been thinking about doing for the previous years since the abortion. Imagine rocking the baby and caring for it and allow yourself to feel love for your baby. You must let the child live, for the moment, so you can identify and have a relationship with your baby.

Again, if you feel comfortable writing, you may want to try writing a letter to your baby, telling him (her) how you feel about the abortion, how you feel about him, how you feel sorry for what you have done. Tell the baby what you would do for him if he were in your arms right now: cradle, love, and talk to him.

Once the baby is alive and real in your mind, it is time to let the baby die. According to Selby, "The baby is dead physically but the post-aborted woman has not allowed the baby to die in her mind. She's only allowed the trauma to exist. So now we allow the grieving to continue or to begin so the baby does die."[13]

---

[12]Terry L. Selby, M.S.W., "Post Abortion Counseling Techniques," presented at Healing Visions, the First National Conference on Post Abortion Counseling, University of Notre Dame (August, 12, 1986), taped lecture.
[13]Ibid., taped lecture.

At this point, Selby suggests that you may want to write out a funeral service for your dead child, again, so you acknowledge that your child is dead and can visualize the actual death.

Whether it is through a service or words you write on paper in a letter to your child, or even verbalizing your thoughts, you need to say goodbye to the baby and your former relationship to it. Express regrets, resentments, and appreciations. By letting your baby die, you are letting go of the effect of the abortion on you. What you retain is your positive remembrance of the baby: his beauty, his love for you, his physical appearance, and whatever qualities you have decided he holds.[14]

Once you've accepted the death of your child, your grieving can begin. You have experienced a loss and you have the need to grieve. In the following chapters we will look at the specific work that needs to be done.

[14]Nancy B. Buckles, M.S., A.C.S.W., "Abortion: A Technique for Working Through Grief," *College Health* (February 1982), p. 181.

CHAPTER FIVE

GUILT AND ANGER

Robin felt worthless. As an unmarried 18-year-old, she faced an unplanned pregnancy. She didn't want to marry the baby's father or give birth to the baby only to relinquish it for adoption. Unemployed and living at home, her future looked bleak. She asked her doctor to recommend an unwed mother's home, where she could live until giving birth. She had decided that her best option was to keep the baby, raising it in her parents' home while she worked. But the doctor said, "Why do you want to do that?" Instead, he recommended that she have an abortion.

Because Robin's pregnancy occurred 17 years ago, before the Supreme Court's *Roe* v. *Wade* decision legalized abortion throughout the United States, she didn't understand what abortion entailed. Her doctor didn't explain the baby's development to her, or what the abortion procedure involved, and she was too afraid to ask. Secretly, Robin feared the pain of childbirth and did not want to be pregnant. After several weeks of struggling with the question of abortion, Robin listened to the advice of her social worker, who told her, "This is what you have to do."

Robin shared her abortion plans with her parents, who attempted to talk her out of the procedure. They didn't tell her that she would be taking a human life or talk in terms of her carrying a baby; they told her she was making a bad decision and they could not support her in this action.

Sixteen weeks into her pregnancy, Robin submitted to a painful saline abortion. All day she waited alone in a hospital room for something to happen, not knowing what to expect. Nothing happened; the abortion attempt failed. Four days later the doctor performed a successful D + E (dilation and evacuation).[1]

After the abortion, Robin's father didn't want anything to do with her. Again, Robin felt worthless. "I had a very low self-esteem before the abortion. The procedure, as well as my father's rejection, compounded my worthlessness." After two unsuccessful months of trying to feel accepted by her parents, Robin moved to be with friends in another state. She supposed a new environment would help her forget the abortion. "But every day the memory of what I had done haunted me. A little voice whispered in my ear: 'Abortion, abortion; you're a terrible, awful person.' "

Although Robin attempted to escape the memory of her abortion, she couldn't escape the guilt.

Guilt is a normal reaction that usually surfaces after the woman recognizes that abortion is wrong and that she is responsible for committing her own abortion. She may

---

[1]In a D & E procedure, the abortionist inserts a pliers-like instrument into the uterus, seizes a leg or other body part, and, with a twisting motion, tears it from the baby's body. Parts that are too large to be removed intact are crushed within the uterus. The process is repeated until all body parts have been removed. Dr. & Mrs. J.C. Willke, *Abortion Questions & Answers* (Cincinnati, Ohio: Hayes Publishing Company, Inc., 1985), p. 85.

feel guilty for one or more reasons: she based her decision on her own self-centered desires; she valued her life more than the life of her child; and/or she committed a sin that went against all moral values. She may feel so guilty and so ashamed that she reasons there is no possible or deserved recovery.

Who experiences guilt?

According to psychological researchers Illsey and Hall, guilt and abortion have become synonymous.[2] No matter what her reason for her abortion, the woman will feel guilt to some degree, whether for a few hours after the procedure is performed or for many years. Some women may not feel guilt immediately, but eventually will. Perhaps she sees a child the same age her aborted baby would have been. Or she becomes pregnant again and decides to keep the baby. This time, she studies fetal development and learns how developed her first baby was when she aborted. Then it hits her, "I killed my baby."

In a survey of aborted women who had experienced stress, 92% of the women reported feelings of guilt.[3] And 35% of the women in another survey listed guilt as their most severe reaction to their abortion experience.[4] Numerous other surveys support this theory of abortion guilt, with a severe guilt reaction occurring in 16%–25% of the women interviewed.[5]

---

[2]R. Illsey and M. Hall, "Psychosocial Research in Abortion: Selected Issues," *Abortion in Psychosocial Perspective: Trends in Transnational Research* (New York: Springer, 1978), pp. 11–34.

[3]Dr. Anne Speckhard, "The Psycho-Social Aspects of Stress Following Abortion," Doctoral Thesis submitted to the University of Minnesota (May 1985), p. 92.

[4]David C. Reardon, preliminary results of a survey of 230 aborted women, basis for his book: *Aborted Women, Silent No More* (Chicago, Ill.: Loyola University Press, 1987).

[5]Dr. Vincent Rue, "Post Abortion Syndrome," presented at Healing Visions, the First National Conference on Post Abortion Counseling, University of Notre Dame (August 11, 1986), p. 11.

Why she experiences guilt

A woman's environment (her family, friends, moral and religious values) will determine if and how much guilt she will experience. For example, a woman is not likely to share her pregnancy or discuss having an abortion with her family if they believe that abortion is wrong. She may fear upsetting her parents and would rather suffer the guilt of an abortion than disappoint them with an unplanned pregnancy. She is, in actuality, protecting her family from having to deal with an issue (abortion) that has already been determined to be wrong. The daughter believes that she must honor an established family belief, so she arranges the abortion secretly and attempts to continue her life as if nothing has happened.

The set of beliefs that a family honors is called the "family paradigm." The beliefs have been developed and shared by the family over the course of their history together. While the beliefs are supported by the family as a whole, a member may not agree on each individual belief. So when a female becomes pregnant in families that oppose out-of-wedlock sex, the decision to abort includes a consideration of whether or not her family can survive a challenge to its belief that out-of-wedlock sex is wrong if she reveals her pregnancy.

A study of stress after abortion revealed that individuals often decided to abort to protect the family paradigm from stress and thus protect their membership in the family, at the cost of their own increased stress.[6]

Mona, pregnant with her lover's child while still married to her husband, had an abortion. Her husband's sterility made it impossible for her to claim the baby was his. She couldn't tell her family, especially her parents, about the affair because such action would not be condoned.

---

[6]Speckhard, op. cit., p. 137.

Years before, Mona had broken the family's rule about premarital sex and had been forced to get married. Now Mona feared that if she told her parents about her pregnancy by her lover, she would be totally rejected by them. Instead, she chose to have the abortion and suffer the consequences, including the guilt that still afflicts her.

Sometimes the woman will not openly share her pregnancy or abortion experience with her parents in order to protect the family paradigm, but she suspects that they know. By not talking about the "secret," the woman protects her family from facing it. A study on the effects of stress on women who have had abortions found that many subjects never told their parents about the abortion (40%), but said that they were quite sure that their parents knew about it or at least suspected it.[7]

Sometimes a woman will feel so guilty about her abortion that she attempts to punish herself for what she has done. According to PAS psychologist Dr. Vincent Rue, "The abortion experience transforms their life into an endless crucifixion of themselves. It is as if they become martyrs, neurotically bidding the will of others with no consideration for their own welfare."[8]

This has happened with Mona, who admits that she is a martyr to her parents. "Their approval means everything to me. They make me feel guilty for not working more (at the family business) and I often wonder, 'What will they think of me because I'm not devoting my life to their company?' I know when they're older that I'll be the one to take care of them. I can't stand their rejection. I can't stand the way I'm living now either. I go home and cry every night; I don't know how to get out of this situation. I'm afraid I'll lose my parents if I don't keep working for them."

---

[7] Ibid., p. 137.
[8] Rue, op. cit., p. 31.

Dr. Rue concludes, "For those who pre-abortion had a marginal self-image, the abortion did nothing to better one's self perception. It did the opposite, and because of the guilt and shame involved, self-alienation and rejection became typical."[9]

Jennifer felt stupid for getting pregnant and helpless because abortion seemed her only alternative. "Immediately after the abortion, the thought kept going through my mind that I was a murderer. I was ashamed, sad, and depressed."

Guilt expressed through anger

Guilt and shame are often expressed through anger. Maureen was enraged at the doctor and nurses who performed her abortion 17 years ago. They did nothing to help her or discourage her abortion. In fact, once on the table being prepared for the abortion, she began sobbing and wanted to leave. "But they forced me down and tied my arms and legs down so I couldn't move."

She is especially angry with the father of the baby, whom she married one month after the abortion. "Now I feel nothing but contempt for my ex-husband. I scream within whenever he's around me."

Maureen is angry with her ex-husband because he did not support her in the pregnancy. Even though they had already planned their church wedding, neither of them wanted the label of "having to get married." According to Maureen, her fiance especially feared his parents' disapproval. She believes he never really wanted her to have children and proved it by his lack of support in her two later pregnancies. He even suggested an abortion during one of those pregnancies because they were experiencing

---

[9]Ibid., p. 32.

marital problems at that time. Now divorced, Maureen feels both anger and sadness towards him.

What causes anger?

For the woman who aborted, anger usually occurs once she realizes that she aborted not "a mass of tissue" but a tiny human being complete with fingers and toes and a heart that really works. Once she has broken the denial that she killed a human life and did not just "end a pregnancy," she is hit with the reality of her decision. As Sandi said upon seeing models of the developing fetus at a right-to-life program, "I walked into that church and saw the fetal models lined up on the table and I realized what I had done. I started crying and wondered where those models were when I was in the abortion clinic."

Dr. Anne Speckhard found in her research of women who aborted that an increased knowledge of fetal development and the methods used to abort the fetus caused a great deal of guilt, anger, and depression, resulting in higher stress. "For some subjects it also caused a degree of concern (and anger) over what they had been told at the abortion facility concerning the fetus (i.e., that it was not a life, that it was a "blob," that it was "only a bunch of cells," etc.)."[10]

Whom is anger directed at?

The anger the woman feels is directed either at people or the event itself. She is especially angry that she got pregnant. "This can't happen to me" is a common statement made when a woman discovers her pregnancy. She may have thought that abortion was her only alternative

---

[10]Speckhard, op. cit., p. 110.

and she is angry that she felt forced to have the abortion. After the abortion, she may be angry that it did indeed happen to her and that now she is just another statistic.

After suffering through the procedure, the woman may be angry, as Maureen was, that she was subjected to such pain and humiliation. She may be angry at her doctor for telling her there would be little pain or complications, when in reality she suffered greatly and experienced any of numerous physical effects. She may have bled for several weeks or contracted a vaginal infection from the instruments used by the doctor. Or an infection may have led to the removal of her uterus.

Anger is also directed at the people involved in the woman's abortion decision: her parents, the baby's father, a friend, or the people at the abortion clinic or doctor's office. They told her that abortion was the only alternative and she believed them. Now she realizes there are other alternatives and it is too late. She may also be angry at them for not having been there for her physically, emotionally or financially. She may even have the subconscious thought that they robbed her of her baby.

According to psychologist Dr. Vincent Rue, anger may be directed at women who never become pregnant or toward those who are happily pregnant and carrying to term, because they haven't had to suffer from abortion. "Some women, post abortion, report feelings of wishing to kidnap children."[11] They want to replace the baby that they believe was stolen from them through abortion.

Abortion sometimes increases bitterness toward men.[12] After all, a man got the woman pregnant and forced her into the situation of having an abortion. Fathers who are aware of the pregnancy often threaten to disown her

---

[11]Rue, op. cit., p. 30.
[12]Ibid., p. 6.

unless she has the abortion. Usually, it is a male doctor who performs the abortion. So when the woman views the whole picture, men seem to be at the base of all her problems and she vents her anger toward them.

This bitterness toward men in general could affect the woman's interactions with people throughout her life. Sandi had three abortions by the time she was 22 years old. "After my abortions, I became more sexually active and promiscuous. But, deep down, I began to hate men."

Besides her hatred for men, Sandi felt an intense hatred for children. She never wanted to give birth and raise a child, so she had a tubal ligation at the age of 25 to prevent herself from ever becoming pregnant again.

The woman's anger can also be directed at the world for the injustice of abortion, anger at God for allowing the pregnancy and the abortion to occur, and anger at the unborn baby for being conceived.[13]

The woman also may be angry with her other children; they survived but her aborted baby did not. Perhaps she had justified her abortion by reasoning that another baby would mean less toys or fewer vacations for the children already born. Or another mouth to feed seemed like an impossibility at the time. But now the guilt of knowing she has killed her child far outweighs any material goods. And she is angry that the four children she does have to feed are here when the fifth one never had a chance to receive her love and care.

Anger may be directed at the pro-life movement for not being available when the woman needed help. Or she might be angry because the pro-life voice forced her to think about the abortion issue, instead of letting her convince herself she had no other choice.

Her anger may be directed at the counselor she turns

---

[13]Ibid., p. 30.

to after the abortion, because he or she represents the group of people who should have helped her when she was pregnant and didn't know what to do. Instead, she relied upon the only option her doctor told her about. Now she realizes that there was accessible help for her.

Lastly, the woman is angry with herself. She is angry because she has allowed her unborn child to be killed and she didn't try to save it. She is angry because she was such a weak person. She couldn't say no when her mother told her she had no other choice. She is angry because she believed the doctor who said she would feel such relief after it was all over and she could start a new life. She is angry because she is alive and her baby isn't.

Anger directed within, according to Dr. Rue, is seen in the forms of self-blame, self-hatred, and shame. "This inner rage may turn to depression, violence, and/or self-destruction."[14]

Deb has experienced anger with herself for not being a stronger person and able to prevent her four aborted pregnancies. She wishes she could have gone to her parents for help or sought alternatives other than abortion. She blames her self-centeredness for leading her into a life of drugs and promiscuity. "By the time I had my fourth abortion, I hated myself. All self-respect was gone. Even though I was married at the time of the last three abortions, I couldn't see myself having a baby and being a mother, subjecting a baby to my shallowness. I recognized my weaknesses and I hated myself for being that way."

Is it OK to get angry?

Anger, whether directed at other people or at oneself, is a normal reaction experienced by the woman who has

---

[14]Ibid., pp. 30–31.

had an abortion. In fact, she needs to express anger if she is to regain her mental and emotional stability. A woman often experiences anger as part of the process of recognizing her personal responsibility for the abortion. As the woman breaks through the denial of her abortion, the full impact of her actions becomes clear. Then she should allow herself the freedom to verbally express her own self-hatred as well as her anger at the social system that supported her actions.[15]

However, anger can be destructive if it is not channeled appropriately. Unresolved anger can cause psychological problems, including depression, impulsive emotional outbursts, aggressive behavior, and sleep problems. Other problems that might develop include sexual dysfunctions, an inability to maintain an intimate relationship, and social isolation.[16]

If you've had an abortion

Perhaps you are angry with someone who influenced your decision to have an abortion. Your anger may be consuming your everyday decision-making ability or it may be simmering just below your apparent composure. Or, you may not even realize you are angry at anyone in particular, yet you sense an inner unrest.

You can be freed from your anger. The first step is to be aware of your anger and desire to get rid of it. You may realize that you have angry feelings about your abortion, but you may not be aware of whom the anger is directed against. So first list all the people who were involved in your abortion decision: the father of the child, your par-

---

[15]Terry L. Selby, M.S.W., "Post Abortion Trauma," unpublished paper, copyright 1984, p. 7. Copy may be obtained by contacting Counseling Associates of Bemidji, Inc., P.O. Box 577, Bemidji, MN 56601.
[16]Ibid., p. 7.

ents, your doctor, counselors at the abortion clinic, your dead baby, and yourself.

Write a letter to each of these persons whom you feel anger against. This is not a letter you will be sending to them; it is simply a means for you to express your feelings. You might begin your letter with this sentence: "I am angry with you because . . ." Be specific about your anger and their actions. If what you write makes you sad and you begin to cry, you will need to rewrite that part. Focus only on your angry feelings. If you find yourself getting away from the subject of anger, go back to your original statement, "I am angry with you because . . ." and concentrate on your angry feelings.

Another exercise used by therapists when counseling women suffering from PAS is to role play.[17] You may not feel comfortable with this technique, but it is a device to make the abstract matter of forgiveness more concrete.

First, set up two chairs, one for the person you are angry at and one for yourself. You can put a pillow or inanimate object in the other chair to represent the person you will be addressing. Talk to that person, preferably out loud, telling him why you are angry with him and what he did to hurt you.

Then trade chairs and pretend you are the other person. Respond as that person would to what you have just said to him. After you've replied, as the other person, move back to your original chair.

Now bring in a third chair, which will be for Jesus Christ. Envision our Savior sitting in the chair looking directly at you. What do you see? How does He look? Once you can see Him in detail, tell Him about your anger for the person in the other chair. Ask Him to help you to get

---

[17]Dr. Anne Speckhard, presentation entitled "Diagnosis and Treatment of Post Abortion Syndrome," given June 18, 1987, at Trinity Lutheran Church in Cedar Rapids, IA.

rid of that anger. How do you think Jesus will reply? Sit in His chair and say what you think He would say. He probably would say, "You must get rid of your anger. You must forgive this person for his part in your abortion, as I have forgiven you. Give me your anger. Let it go; I will bear it for you."

With God's help, you will be able to forgive the person or people you are angry with. This will not happen overnight; you must pray for strength and wisdom daily and work at forgiving them. The other person can't bring your dead baby back to life, so no amount of anger will make up for your loss. Leave injustices in God's hands and set yourself free. "Do not take revenge, my friends, but leave room for God's wrath, for it is written: 'It is mine to avenge; I will repay,' says the Lord" (Rom. 12:19).

CHAPTER SIX

BARGAINING, DEPRESSION AND ISOLATION, FEAR

Once the woman experiences guilt and anger, she realizes that abortion isn't the easy choice she thought it would be. Instead, abortion has brought her emotional pain that she never knew she could feel.

To rationalize her pain, she reminds herself, "Abortion was my only choice. I didn't want to do it but I had to. And I know it's something I'll never do again."

BARGAINING

Comments like these are commonly spoken by women in the post-abortion stage known as bargaining. When the aborted woman is in the bargaining phase, she will say and do things hoping to stop the grieving process. She may throw herself into various activities, such as her job, so that she has no time or energy left to face the continued reality of her grief.[1]

Another way that she may bargain her abortion is to

---

[1]Terry L. Selby, M.S.W., "Post Abortion Trauma," unpublished paper, copyright 1984, p. 8. Copy may be obtained by contacting Counseling Associates of Bemidji, Inc., P.O. Box 577, Bemidji, MN 56601.

have another baby to compensate for the baby she aborted. By becoming pregnant, she convinces herself that this is the baby she lost. Or she might try to become a "super-mom" to her other children, leading every group they belong to, always cleaning up after them at home, working outside the home just to provide their material desires, and, in general, giving them whatever they want.

Or the woman who bargains her abortion may become active in a crisis pregnancy center or speak out against abortion before she has been honest with herself about her own abortion. She rationalizes that she is helping women by providing them with the facts of abortion, but inside she believes that she is making up or "paying her dues" for the abortion she has had. "If I speak enough times," she thinks, "then that will make up for my abortion—it will help erase what I've done."

One problem with this thinking, according to Dr. Anne Speckhard, is that it only delays dealing with the reality of what she did when she had the abortion. If she carries a later pregnancy to term, the reality of what she did to her first baby surfaces and she has to cope with her abortion at that point. Also, the sex of the second baby may not be the sex of the baby she aborted and/or thought she would have had. Then she can't view the baby as the one she aborted. The baby is a unique and separate individual, and so she must then deal with the first one and how he died.[2]

Carol is in her ninth month of pregnancy and has had three abortions. She told her sister that she never thought of her other pregnancies as actual babies, that they were like having the flu and the abortions were the cure. Her sister, who regrets her own abortion, is concerned that the

---

[2]Dr. Anne Speckhard, presentation entitled "Diagnosis and Treatment of Post Abortion Syndrome," given June 18, 1987, at Trinity Lutheran Church in Cedar Rapids, Iowa.

birth of the baby will force Carol to deal with her earlier abortions. "I hope she doesn't have any problems over the past when her baby is born. When your baby is born, you feel such a strong love for it that it almost hurts. I just hope she can put the past behind her. She doesn't talk much about it, but there was something in her voice [when she talked about her abortions] that I sensed she was dealing with some strong emotions."

When a woman bargains her abortion, she doesn't have to deal with the pain of grief and guilt. But once the barriers created by bargaining are down, she is likely to experience depression. Because the bargaining phase is based on the idea that she can reconcile her grief through super-human deeds, which in reality cannot be accomplished, she *will* fail. It is her failure that leads her back to a state of emotional upset that is the beginning of depression.[3]

If you've had an abortion

Do you suspect that you've been bargaining your abortion? You may have told yourself that abortion is wrong but, in your case, it had to be done. Or you feel compelled to speak about your experience at pro-life meetings, not because you want to inform others about the realities of abortion but because it makes you feel good, and somehow your abortion seems justified.

Examine your feelings about your abortion experience:

1. Do you blame people or your personal situation as the cause of your abortion? If you believe that your abortion was the result more of outside factors than your own action, then you are still employing a form of denial. To break this denial of your role in the abortion, consider

---

[3]Selby, op. cit., p. 8.

how you could have prevented it. At what point could you have said, "I won't allow this abortion to happen."

2. Have you admitted to yourself and to God that what you did was wrong? Focus on your own individual personality. Examine your weaknesses and recognize that you made a mistake. Then thank God for loving you as you are and offering to you the forgiveness and peace that you so desperately need.

DEPRESSION AND ISOLATION

When a woman realizes that her abortion was a terminal and unchangeable act, she will become depressed. Her pain and suffering may show up in physical problems (such as back pain or headaches), weight loss, alcohol and drug abuse, psychological problems (ranging from unexpected emotional outbursts and low self-esteem to thoughts of suicide), and social, family, and other relational problems. She is typical in this phase if she feels she is an unforgivable person. In her mind, she has committed the worst possible sin and sees no way to make up for what she has done.[4]

Julie was 17 years old and six-to-eight weeks pregnant when she had her abortion. She couldn't marry the father because he was in the United States on a student visa and his family would not permit it. As the eldest of four children, Julie felt expected to achieve, to graduate from high school and go on to college and a career. She couldn't raise a baby herself. She tried to find a facility where she could live until the baby was born and then give it up for adoption, but at the time of her pregnancy, these resources were not readily available. Her parents were very coercive and told her that abortion was the only answer. It seemed

---

[4]Ibid., pp. 9–10.

so hopeless that Julie finally agreed to the abortion, even though as a Christian, she knew it was morally wrong. Afterward, she struggled with her Christian walk. "I fluctuated between feeling like hell should open up and swallow me, and knowing I can be forgiven. But then I would wonder, 'How can I deserve to be forgiven?' I think I asked for forgiveness 800 times, but I never felt like I could be really forgiven. I felt awful and when I asked for forgiveness, the feeling didn't go away."

There is no time limit on depression. A woman may function in this stage only for a short while, or for years. How long depends on when she recognizes that she is in a state of depression and seeks professional counseling or attempts to help herself overcome her depression.

Also, her depression may be delayed for several years. She may not recognize the significance of her abortions until she later experiences periods of emotional depression. When counseling women in their 50's and 60's for depression, psychiatrists frequently hear thoughts of remorse and guilt concerning abortions that were performed 20 or more years earlier.[5] Also, women who undergo legal abortion may develop, even years later, numerous emotional disorders that will reach a climax when menopause occurs.[6]

Who becomes depressed?

The studies the author reviewed showed depression to be the most common effect experienced by women post-abortion. One study of 2,771 aborters showed that the most common psychological disturbances were "depres-

---

[5] Dr. Anne Speckhard, "The Psycho-Social Aspects of Stress Following Abortion," Doctoral Thesis submitted to the University of Minnesota (May 1985), p. 16.
[6] Ibid., p. 17.

sive personality developments with self-accusation and guilt complexes, fears of infertility, sexual phobias and other symptoms resulting from unresolved conflicts." In another study of 30 women who had high stress abortion experiences, feelings of depression were experienced by 92% of the subjects. Also, 69% reported feelings of hopelessness and helplessness.[7]

How does a woman know if she is in a state of depression? A woman suffering from post-abortion depression does not care about herself and is lethargic.[8] She may experience a number of changes, such as emotional numbness, feelings of worthlessness, dependence on drugs and alcohol, new behavior relating to her sexuality, preoccupation with the aborted child, isolation and alienation, and thoughts of suicide.

Emotional numbness

At this point, the woman may feel like an emotional cripple. She has shut down her emotions and won't let herself feel anything.[9]

In the study of 30 women having experienced a high-stress abortion, suppressing emotions in order to cope was a common reaction. In fact, 73% of the women reported the inability to experience emotions, particularly painful emotions, after the abortion. Terms used to describe this experience were numbness or shock, an inability to feel emotions, repression, and a shutting down of feelings.[10]

---

[7] Ibid., p. 88.

[8] Dr. Anne Speckhard, presentation entitled "Diagnosis and Treatment of Post Abortion Syndrome," given June 18, 1987, at Trinity Lutheran Church in Cedar Rapids, Iowa.

[9] Ibid.

[10] Dr. Anne Speckhard, "The Psycho-Social Aspects of Stress Following Abortion," Doctoral Thesis submitted to the University of Minnesota (May 1985), p. 83.

Mona had her abortion eight years ago and still feels the emotional effects of the procedure. "I feel like I am a colder person now. I'm numb where I use to be so vulnerable. I used to grieve for dead babies or hurt children. Now there is nothing. I don't want to hurt like that again, where I grieve for a hurting child."

Many women, particularly teenagers, seem to be unaffected by an induced abortion. They might even brag, "I've had three abortions and they haven't affected me." But some psychiatrists (Kent, 1977) believe this type of emotional numbness, which appears to be positive, is really an adverse reaction, requiring psychiatric attention.[11] Many of the subjects who suffered from a high-stress abortion were able to suppress the effects of their abortion until future fertility issues were confronted. Just seeing other pregnant women or small children often caused feelings of guilt or grief. Increased painful emotions often accompanied menstruation. Conception after the abortion was a stressful time for many of the subjects. If they failed to conceive or suffered a miscarriage, they believed it was a result of their abortion and felt guilty for having caused a second terminated pregnancy.[12]

According to Dr. Vincent Rue, the realization of abortion death leaves the parent dazed and out of step with life and the meaning of relationships. "Guilt and grief are solitary. Hence, we do not choose whether or not we should be guilty or grieve—we just do. Many individuals at this point feel less a person, less integrated, less able to function, less able to make decisions and judgments, and so self-negative as to despair of life itself. Their bodies hurt, aching with emptiness, fatigue and guilt, for which there is no rest. They may not be able to sleep or may find

---

[11]Ibid., p. 17.
[12]Speckhard, op. cit., p. 151.

excessive sleep an escape. Nightmares and dreams of the child that never was are common, leaving one filled with remorse and exhaustion. Wishes for the undoing of the death of the child may engage one's imagination, creating the image, the voice, the touch, and the footsteps that never were. Madness can be fantasized as relief."[13]

Feelings of worthlessness

For the woman who is emotionally immature, the consequences of abortion deepen her feelings of inferiority, inadequacy, insignificance, and worthlessness. Society tells her that she has a right to control her own body, that abortion is a simple, safe procedure, that she should exercise her right to choose, and that she is justified in not exposing an unwanted child to the trauma of being unloved. According to psychiatrist Dr. Conrad W. Baars, "The bitter realization that she was not even unselfish enough to share her life with another human being will take its toll. If she had ever entertained a doubt as to whether her parents and others really considered her unlovable and worthless, she will now be certain that she was indeed never any good in their eyes or her own. A deep depression will be inevitable and her preoccupation with thoughts of suicide that much greater."[14]

Drugs and alcohol

Some women choose to suppress the effects of abortion through the increased use of drugs and alcohol. 61%

---

[13]Dr. Vincent M. Rue, "Post Abortion Syndrome," presented at Healing Visions, the First National Conference on Post Abortion Counseling, University of Notre Dame (August 11, 1986), p. 29.

[14]Conrad W. Baars, M.D., "Psychic Causes and Consequences of the Abortion Mentality," *The Psychological Aspects of Abortion* (Washington, D.C.: University Publications of America, Inc., 1979), pp. 121–122.

of the 30 women who suffered high-stress abortion experiences reported increased use of alcohol, and 58% reported increased use of drugs (both licit and illicit). 50% of the subjects reported patterns of drug or alcohol addiction after the abortion. The majority of subjects reported that their first heavy drug and alcohol use occurred as a result of the stress related to abortion. Only three subjects stated that they had already developed an unhealthy reliance on drugs and alcohol as a means of coping prior to the abortion.[15]

Deb found relief from her abortion guilt through alcohol and drugs, which were readily available through her husband, a drug dealer. "After my fourth abortion, I was still doing drugs and hated myself for what I had done. I had no self-respect and couldn't see myself having a baby and being a mother."

Sexuality

A woman's sexuality is also likely to be affected by her abortion. Some post-abortion women find themselves wanting sex more often, attempting to become pregnant to fill the emptiness or looking for partners for casual sex in a desperate attempt to find relief and acceptance. Other women lose all libido and detest the slightest sexual touch, remembering how their aborted pregnancy began, and fearing the possibility of pregnancy and more suffering.[16]

How many women experience sexuality problems post-abortion? In the study of 30 women who suffered high-stress abortions, feelings of sexual inhibition after the abortion were reported by 69% of the women. 35% of

---

[15]Speckhard, op. cit., p. 84.
[16]Rue, op. cit., p. 30.

the subjects listed sexual anxiety. According to the researcher, Dr. Anne Speckhard, "Feelings of sexual anxiety and inhibition appeared to be linked to feelings of guilt and anxiety regarding the potential for another pregnancy. Although feelings of sexual anxiety were reported to cause a decrease in pleasure in the sexual relationship, such feelings did not in all cases cause sexual inhibition as well."[17]

At the other end of the spectrum, 31% of the subjects reported sexual promiscuity following abortion. The subjects defined sexual promiscuity as having many sexual partners, as opposed to one or none, within a defined period of time.[18]

After her four abortions, the last three of which were done during her first marriage, Deb found herself having casual sexual relationships with men she really didn't care about. "Satan knew my weak point and it was men."

After every relationship, Deb would experience a crushing feeling that her world was caving in and she would think about the abortions. "I was going through a horrible mental torment; I would go home at night and drink obnoxious amounts of alcohol and go lay in the bathtub with a candle burning. I could feel this horrible battle going on."

Another reaction is the effect on the sexual relationship with the father of the baby. In the same study of 30 women, it was found that in cases where the relationship continued past the abortion, 35% of the subjects reported a deterioration in the sexual relationship. Increased sexual anxiety and inhibitions relating to guilt and fear of another pregnancy were given as reasons for this problem. In many cases the relationships themselves were deteriorating, which contributed to the decreased pleasure in

---

[17]Speckhard, op. cit., p. 78.
[18]Ibid., p. 78.

the sexual part of the relationship.[19]

In another study of 230 women, 10% reported experiencing sexual coldness or revulsion of sex following their abortions. Also, 30% listed depression and 20% listed lowered self-worth or self-esteem as the most severe reaction to their abortion.[20]

Preoccupation with the child

The woman post-abortion is often preoccupied with the characteristics of her aborted child. This reaction, reported in 81% of the subjects in the study of high-stress aborters, was revealed in many ways, with the most common response focusing on the date the child would have been born and the age it would be at subsequent "birthdays." Some women wondered about the sex, eye and hair coloring, and height of the child, if it had been born. The periods of preoccupation were highest on anniversary dates, including the date of the abortion and the pregnancy due date. Preoccupation with the aborted child also occurred immediately after the abortion, especially if the woman saw another infant or small child.[21]

Isolation, alienation

The woman may feel isolated from the rest of the everyday world. Elections are held and seasons change, but she feels out of touch with reality. She seems to exist from day to day, with no meaning to her life. This avoidance phenomena can show up in any of the following ways:

---

[19]Ibid., p. 79.
[20]David Reardon, *Aborted Women, Silent No More* (Chicago, IL: Loyola University Press, 1987).
[21]Speckhard, op. cit., p. 89.

1. She feels a distinctly diminished interest in significant activities.

2. She feels detached from friends and relatives.

3. Her capacity for feeling or expressing emotions is less than normal.

4. She communicates less verbally and/or experiences hostile encounters with other people.

5. She feels she is in a depressed mood.[22]

How common is this feeling of isolation? In the study of high-stress aborters, 69% of the sample reported increased feelings of loneliness, isolation, and alienation following the abortion. This was often related to the inability to discuss the abortion with others. In nearly half the cases, the relationship with the father of the baby ended and, because the male partner was often the only other person who knew about the abortion, this created a large void in the woman's life. This contributed to feelings of loneliness, isolation, and alienation.[23]

Suicide

The woman who commits suicide post-abortion may be rare, but the number who entertain suicidal thoughts is not so rare. One study shows that 12% of the women had suicidal thoughts, with 3% attempting suicide. And women who were counseled as psychiatric patients before the abortion were three times as likely to require therapy after the abortion.[24]

A woman becomes very hardened and despairing, considering suicide, because she has tried to work out her problems, including an unplanned pregnancy, but she

---

[22]Rue, op. cit., p. 36.

[23]Speckhard, op. cit., p. 86.

[24]Dr. Vincent M. Rue, "Abortion in Relationship Context," International Review of Natural Family Planning, Summer (1985): 113.

doesn't see any change in her emotional well-being. As her depression continues for months and then years, she cares less and less about herself and views suicide as her only way out of the pain and lack of meaning in life.[25]

In the study of high-stress aborters, 65% of the subjects reported having suicidal thoughts as a reaction to the abortion experience, and 31% of the women actually made suicide attempts. Suicidal thoughts were most often reported as having self-destructive thoughts that were never translated into concrete actions. Suicide attempts were in most cases drug and/or alcohol overdoses that resulted in hospitalization.[26]

Nancyjo's abortion during her fifth month of pregnancy led her to a drug and alcohol dependency as well as a promiscuous lifestyle. All were attempts to block the painful memory of her saline abortion, which haunted her.

One cold January night, in desperation, Nancyjo turned to a bottle of barbiturates. Many times she had considered killing herself but had always stopped. She wasn't sure why. But this time she intended to do it. She had nothing to live for—no hope of any kind. She couldn't stay high forever nor support her expensive drug habit.

Then, for some reason unknown to Nancyjo, she turned to a copy of The Living Bible that her mother had given her that previous Christmas. She didn't know what the Bible even had to offer, but it seemed to call to her, to open its cover. "I looked in the Bible and read some passages, but it didn't make any sense to me," Nancyjo said. "I just cried, 'Please, God, give me a reason to live.' " With

---

[25]Dr. Anne Speckhard, presentation entitled "Diagnosis and Treatment of Post Abortion Syndrome," given June 18, 1987, at Trinity Lutheran Church in Cedar Rapids, Iowa.

[26]Dr. Anne Speckhard, "The Psycho-Social Aspects of Stress Following Abortion," Doctoral Thesis submitted to the University of Minnesota (May 1985), pp. 87–88.

that prayer, Nancyjo flushed the pills down the toilet, and, exhausted, fell asleep on her bed with the Bible clutched to her breast.

Suicide prevention groups are finding a relation with post-abortion women and suicide attempts or thoughts of suicide. The Ohio Regional Director of Suiciders Anonymous reported that out of the 4,000 women with whom the group had contact during a 35-month period, 1,800, or 45%, of the women had had abortions.[27]

The woman who has had multiple abortions is more likely to consider suicide and to be depressed. 40% of the 71 women studied reported anniversary reactions on the date of the abortion, and the expected delivery date of the child would cause an emotional reaction, such as crying, listlessness, and reliving the memory of the abortion experience. Half of the women sought psychotherapy after the abortion.[28]

If you've had an abortion

Do you suspect that you are in a state of depression and isolation because of your abortion? Have you experienced an emotional numbness, worthlessness, dependence on drugs and alcohol, new sexual behavior, preoccupation with your aborted child, or suicidal thoughts?

If so, you need to talk about your abortion experience with someone you trust, someone who will listen to you and not condemn you. If possible, you should talk to a Christian counselor, who can help you through your depression to recovery. If you don't feel comfortable talk-

---

[27]Dennis and Matthew Linn, S.J., and Sheila Fabricant, M. Div., "Healing Relationships with Miscarried, Aborted, and Stillborn Babies," *Journal of Christian Healing* (Vol. 7, No. 2), p. 21.

[28]Dr. Vincent Rue, "Post Abortion Syndrome," presented at Healing Visions, the First National Conference on Post Abortion Counseling, University of Notre Dame (August 11, 1986), p. 14.

ing to a professional counselor, you may want to contact a post-abortion women's group. These groups may be listed in your telephone directory by name (see Appendix C) or they may be connected with a social service agency. Usually, by calling their telephone number, you can talk to someone who has had an abortion experience and will understand what you have been through. If you have a friend you can confide in, you may want to tell him or her what you have been feeling. Just talking out your frustrations and concerns can be a relief. Again, you are the best judge for the type of help you need the most, whether it be just talking to a close friend or seeking professional counseling. Don't believe that the confusion and pain is something you have to handle on your own. There are concerned people waiting to help you, if only you will let them.

FEAR

Post-abortion women may fear a number of things: that others will find out about the abortion, punishment from God, infertility, subsequent pregnancy losses, and loss of dignity.

In the study of high-stress aborters, the percentage of women experiencing fear were as follows:[29]

Fear that others would find out—89%.

General feelings of anxiety—54%.

Fear of punishment by God—50%.

Fear of future infertility—46%.

After two abortions, Jane was angry, confused, and depressed. "I searched for some meaning to life, but I felt empty inside. I would go to parties and try to forget who I was and what I had done. This led to more confusion

---

[29]Speckhard, op. cit., pp. 76–77.

and destruction. I didn't know who I was or what I was doing. I just reached the end of a rope. I was struggling to hang on but didn't know how to do it. I became real fearful. I took myself to the emergency room of the local University Hospital. I thought to myself, *They're going to think I'm crazy, but I need help and I don't know who to turn to.* I had never talked about my abortions to anybody. By that time I was a physical mess; I hadn't been sleeping for four months, plus I was working full time. I didn't want to take care of myself. I was becoming anorexic and didn't care about my health. I thought a lot about the abortions and had no self-worth.

"I pleaded with the people in the emergency room to help me. 'What's the matter?' they asked. 'I really don't know, but I know I need help,' I told them. I thought I might have a blood disease where you get real weak. I asked them to do a blood test, but they didn't find anything wrong. So they examined me and called in a psychiatrist. I pleaded with them to put me into the hospital. I thought there was something physically wrong, but they said I was normal. *Why am I going through all these feelings if I'm normal?* I thought. I was very fearful of myself and didn't trust myself. I thought I might even kill myself. I told the psychiatrist I was scared to go home by myself. He just talked to me and said, 'You know things about your past that bother you.' I didn't tell him about my abortions. I said thanks and went home to my apartment. Only this time I turned to Jesus."

Jane had known about Jesus and had attended church, but it wasn't until that night that she turned to Him for help. When she returned to her apartment, she picked up her Bible and hugged it to her chest, crying and asking Jesus into her life. "At that moment I felt that someone had picked me off the ground, given me a big hug and kiss and said, 'It's going to be all right.' I felt all warm inside, where I had been so cold for a long time.''

If you've had an abortion

Have you been a victim of fear? With God's help, you can rise above your fear. You do have value in God's eyes and are a worthwhile person. Think back to who you were before your abortion. Perhaps you were a teenager, making plans for your senior prom and graduation. Or you were a college student, ready to experience life and all it has to offer. Or maybe you were a mother of three young children, working hard at a full-time job to help pay the bills. Did you feel good about yourself at that time? Did you have a sense of worth? You are still that same person, just a little older and much wiser now. You are still a contributing member of society and have much to offer. You made a mistake, but through God's forgiveness, you can start over and live a meaningful life.

There are some specific steps you can take to help heal your feelings of fear. First, ask Jesus to heal whatever hurts caused you to abort your child. Was it the fear of what other people might think? Or were you a single working woman who didn't want to raise a child alone? Think back to the circumstances surrounding your abortion and consider what factors led you to abortion. Then, turn to Jesus and pray that He heal you of those memories and feelings of inadequacy.

Second, consider the fears that you now have (the fear that others will find out about your abortion, fear of future infertility, fear of punishment). Consider each one that applies to you, carefully looking at the consequences if each fear were to come true. Then, place your fears into God's hands; let Him hold them for you. Know that even if your worst fears were to come true, God would be with you and would take care of you.

Again, if you feel that you need help in overcoming your depression or fear, please contact a Christian counselor. You are not alone in this matter. There are caring Christians who are waiting to help. All you need do is reach out for their help.

CHAPTER SEVEN

FORGIVENESS

In her book *The Ambivalence of Abortion*, Linda Bird Francke recounts her first-trimester abortion in New York City. She and her husband, parents of two daughters, had decided against having a third child. He was in the process of a career change, and the added stress of a new baby would be more than they felt they could handle. In addition, they had planned a long summer vacation that would have to be canceled if they had the baby.

But despite her arguments that the abortion was necessary, Linda reveals that she now lives with remorse that takes the form of a ghost. "A very little ghost," she explains, "that only appears when I'm seeing something beautiful, like the full moon on the ocean last weekend. And the baby waves at me. And I wave at the baby. 'Of course, we have room,' I cry to the ghost. 'Of course, we do.' "[1]

Linda, like many women who abort an unwanted baby, is haunted by the memory of the child she rejected. Her vision may represent regret or perhaps doubt in her "nec-

---

[1]Linda Bird Francke, *The Ambivalence of Abortion* (New York, N.Y.: Random House, Inc., 1978), p. 7.

essary" decision. For other women who have had this same experience, being tormented by their dead baby's ghost is frightening and emotionally crippling. To such a woman, her baby is a real person crying to her from the dead, never to be consoled in his mother's arms.

Sarah is haunted by recurring nightmares about the baby she aborted at 18 weeks. In her dreams, she recalls the horror of her saline abortion. She sees her bloodied lifeless son in a cold metal basin for several minutes before he is taken away to be cremated in the hospital incinerator (symbolizing the burning of her baby's body by the chemicals of her saline abortion).

Then the dream shifts to unreality as the nurse, before taking the baby away, shoves the basin under Sarah's nose and screams, "See what you did, you murderer! You killed your own son! What kind of a mother are you?"

At that point, Sarah awakes, trembling with fear and usually crying, "I didn't want to do it! I didn't want to do it!" She spends the rest of the night in self-condemnation.

Feeling unfit even to live, Sarah often contemplates suicide. She avoids personal relationships with anyone, especially men, and buries herself in her work as a computer programmer. Thin and pale, Sarah does not look well and has lost her will to live.

Not all women who have had abortions experience such extreme symptoms of guilt. For many, there is a growing uneasiness that what they did was wrong. They begin to doubt their ability to be a mother or possess mothering qualities. "How can I be a good mother to one child when I've aborted another?" the woman might ask.

These women are often able to act normally around friends and co-workers, while inside a ball of pain intensifies whenever they see an infant or small child. Some women are afraid to talk to a close friend or spouse about their feelings. Others have even cut off those once intimate relationships. Many women feel all alone in the world and don't like themselves very much, so they can't imagine how anyone else could possibly like her. How can these women get rid of their guilt feelings and become a part of life again? The answer is found in forgiveness.

What is forgiveness?

Forgiveness is the act of absolving a person of his wrongs or sins whereby the guilty person is released both from his guilt and punishment.[2] For the woman who has had an abortion, this means that she is cleared of her abortion, and she, in turn, stops feeling resentment against the people who influenced her abortion decision. No punishment must be endured; the slate is simply wiped clean.

Forgiveness does not just free a woman from her sin; it provides a total deliverance from sin and restores the woman to fellowship with God.[3] "But now a righteousness from God, apart from law, has been made known, to which the Law and the Prophets testify. This righteousness from God comes through faith in Jesus Christ to all who believe. There is no difference, for all have sinned and fall short of the glory of God, and are justified freely by his grace through the redemption that came by Christ Jesus" (Rom. 3:21–24).

Why does the woman who has had an abortion need forgiveness?

The woman needs forgiveness so that she can live the rest of her days on earth in joy and peace. Forgiveness

---

[2]Colin Brown, General Editor, *The New International Dictionary of New Testament Theology* (Grand Rapids, Mich.: Zondervan Publishing House, 1975), Vol. I: A-F, p. 698.
[3]Ibid., p. 702.

allows her to lay down the guilt she has been carrying with her since she first realized that she killed her baby. It lets her start over again.

She needs forgiveness for her own safety. As an unhealed person, that is, unhealed from abortion's emotional aftermath, she has a tremendous capacity to destroy herself. Because she feels guilty for having made the decision to abort her baby, she thinks that she has to punish herself for her sin. In fact, she almost wills herself to be injured so that she has a reason for her suffering. "If I can punish myself physically," she reasons, "then perhaps I will be paying for the abortion."

A woman needs forgiveness because her abortion affects her attitude about other people. She doesn't trust anyone because either her doctor, mother or boyfriend deceived her into thinking that abortion was a clean, easy solution to her problem pregnancy. Now she wonders if anything they tell her is true. If they could deceive her about abortion, then they could deceive her about everything. "They didn't really care about me then," she reasons, "so why should I care about them now?"

She needs forgiveness because what she has done is wrong. Her abortion is an offense against God, the child, and herself. And killing her child through abortion breaks God's laws and the laws of nature.

Although man-made laws condone abortion, it is wrong in God's eyes and breaks the fifth commandment, "You shall not murder" (Ex. 20:13).

Life is precious in God's sight. After all, He is the Creator of all life. He knows each of us before we are born, before we are even conceived, and knows what each day of our life will be like. "Before I formed you in the womb I knew you, before you were born I set you apart" (Jer. 1:5).

Many people insist that the unborn fetus is just a mass

of tissue and not really human because it has no useful value. And because a person's spirit can't be seen entering the body, it's easy to assume that this occurs at birth when the baby appears outside the womb. Some people believe the baby becomes a person at its quickening, when the mother first feels the child moving inside her.

But God has ordained life and given it value even before its conception and birth. "For you created my inmost being; you knit me together in my mother's womb. I praise you because I am fearfully and wonderfully made; your works are wonderful, I know that full well. My frame was not hidden from you when I was made in the secret place. When I was woven together in the depths of the earth, your eyes saw my unformed body. All the days ordained for me were written in your book before one of them came to be" (Ps. 139:13–16).

We can't understand how a body receives a soul because it's beyond our human reasoning; we can only accept it. "As you do not know the path of the wind, or how the body is formed in a mother's womb, so you cannot understand the work of God, the Maker of all things" (Eccles. 11:5).

A life ended through abortion goes against God's desires. The woman, in effect, is saying that the life God created has no value because it happened at an inconvenient time or the gender was wrong or it may not be perfect physically or mentally. She's saying that she knows better than God whether that life should be allowed to continue and serve a purpose.

A woman may say, "I didn't think all of those things when I considered having my abortion. It scared me to think about what a pregnancy and baby would do to my life. And I thought of the baby, because I just couldn't bring it into the world when I had no means to support it and no stable family life."

Look back at those reasons. How many times did she say the word "I"? At the time of her abortion, her feelings were really focused on *her* life, not on the baby's welfare. She could have objected with any number of reasons, but they all would be based on the fact that she placed her own self-interests first, whether to protect herself from someone who said she had to have the abortion or for her own personal reasons. That is a normal reaction in a crisis situation. It is human nature to protect oneself. But when it provides the rationale for an abortion, the new life of the child is devalued and ended.

Besides breaking God's law, aborting one's own child goes against the natural process for which a woman's body is designed. Physically, the female body is designed to conceive and bear children. The unborn child is nurtured and protected in the womb even before the mother is aware of its existence. An abortion stops this natural process of nurturing that the body is prepared to follow and prevents the body from doing its job. It's telling nature, "Sorry, I know the fetus is alive, growing and quickly developing, nurtured by the womb, but I don't want the end result." All the life-sustaining equipment is suddenly shut down and the body is robbed of the new life. For several weeks or months, the body has been taking care of the fetus. Now, quite abruptly and harshly, through abortion, the womb is stripped of its contents.

Forgiveness for eternity

The woman who chose abortion needs to be reconciled to God for her sin so that as a clean, forgiven soul she can enjoy life not only on earth but also for eternity in heaven.

Under God's laws, she has been convicted for her sin. She has been found guilty. It's as if she is serving a sentence for her deed. She feels that sentence every waking hour. She may not always be thinking about the abortion itself, and if she's lucky, she may go for several hours or even all day without an unhappy remembrance. Even then, a heaviness hangs on her, dragging her spirits. Something doesn't seem quite right and she can't shake the feeling.

There is good news for her: she can be released of her guilt through Jesus Christ. The verdict can be lifted. "Therefore, there is no condemnation for those who are in Christ Jesus, because through Christ Jesus, the law of the Spirit of life set me free from the law of sin and death" (Rom. 8:1–2).

If she has been plagued by the image of a baby reaching out to her, and her heart aches to undo the abortion because she can't live with the memory of what she has done, then she can rejoice at the peace that forgiveness in Jesus offers.

How can the woman be forgiven?

Before she can even think of forgiveness, she must believe that God is the Creator of all life and that she ended a life through her abortion. Then she can recognize she needs His forgiveness for what she has done. In humility, she needs to talk to Him, to express her feelings, either silently in her bed at night or aloud in her living room— wherever she feels comfortable. This is communication between her and God. No one else need hear. Wherever she is, God will hear her.

Admitting guilt

When talking to God, the woman should admit her part in taking the life of an unborn child. She can simply say, "I killed my unborn child." But she must believe it in her heart. She could remember the day she had her abortion and how she let the doctor reassure her that she was doing the right thing or how she didn't question the development of her baby. She allowed it to happen, even if she had wanted to stop the procedure in the last moments, but didn't. "Yes, I killed my baby. My friends may have encouraged me, my doctor may have recommended it, but ultimately, it was my decision. I am guilty."

"If we confess our sins, he is faithful and just and will forgive us our sins and purify us from all unrighteousness" (1 John 1:9).

Repentance

After admitting her guilt, the woman should feel sorry for her abortion and admit her sin. She can say, "I am sorry that I killed my baby. I know it was wrong to do. I was selfish. I regret my action." She shouldn't make excuses for her decision or rationalize her action. God knows what they are. Rather, He wants to hear her admit her sorrow for letting circumstances lead her to choose abortion.

Maureen blocked out the memory of her abortion until she was in labor with her daughter. Then she questioned why abortions are allowed. But she really didn't deal with the abortion until several years later, when she began to feel uneasy about life and why things happened, including her divorce. Her awareness that she needed to deal with past events in her life grew after talking to her priest about her inner turmoil. He instructed her to think about her past and recall any events that she may have buried. When she admitted that she had had an abortion, the priest asked her to look even further back to examine what factors had led to the abortion. Then she realized that premarital sex was at the root of the problem, and she needed to repent of that sin as well as the abortion.

Through repentance, a woman accepts God's verdict of sin and prepares her heart for deliverance through forgiveness in Christ Jesus.

Asking God's forgiveness

Once she has repented of her abortion, the woman should specifically ask God to forgive her for killing her unborn child. She might say, "Dear Father, you are the Creator of all life, including my own. Please forgive me for killing a life that you had ordained. I need the peace that only your forgiveness can give me. Please hear my prayer. Amen."

King David was an Old Testament believer who understood the true meaning of forgiveness. After he had committed adultery with Bathsheba, he prayed the verses found in Psalm 51. This prayer could be used by women seeking God's forgiveness by replacing the given words with the words in parenthesis:

"Have mercy on me, O God, according to your unfailing love;

according to your great compassion blot out my transgressions (abortion).

Wash away all my iniquity (sins) and cleanse me from my sin (abortion).

For I know my transgressions, and my sin (abortion) is always before me.

Against you, you only, have I sinned and done what is evil in your sight (by killing my unborn child), so that you are proved right when you speak and justified when you judge (that I have sinned).

Surely I have been a sinner from birth, sinful from the time my mother conceived me.

Surely you desire truth in the inner parts (that I recognize that my abortion was a sin against you); you teach me wisdom in the inmost place.

Cleanse me with hyssop, and I will be clean; wash me, and I will be whiter than snow.

Let me hear joy and gladness; let the bones you have crushed rejoice.

Hide your face from my sins (including abortion) and blot out all my iniquity (sins relating to my abortion).

Create in me a pure heart, O God, and renew a steadfast spirit within me.

Do not cast me from your presence or take your Holy Spirit from me.

Restore to me the joy of your salvation and grant me a willing spirit, to sustain me.

Then I will teach transgressors (other women who chose abortion) your ways, and sinners will turn back to you.

Save me from bloodguilt (the blood shed through my abortion), O God, the God who saves me, and my tongue will sing of your righteousness (I will tell others what you have done for me).

O Lord, open my lips, and my mouth will declare your praise. You do not delight in sacrifice, or I would bring it; you do not take pleasure in burnt offerings.

The sacrifices of God are a broken spirit; a broken and contrite heart (one that admits its abortion was wrong and asks for forgiveness), O God, you will not despise."

———Psalm 51:1–18

Why should God forgive her?

"Why," she might ask, "would God want to forgive me? I'm a terrible person and don't deserve His forgiveness." The good news is, GOD LOVES HER! She is a child of God, too, just as her unborn child is. God wants to forgive her for her sins, and He will if she only admits them and asks for His forgiveness. God hates sin, including abortion, but He loves her, the sinner. God is a loving Father who wraps His arms around her and holds her when she is hurting. He cries with her for the loss of her baby and wants her to feel whole again. "I have loved you with an everlasting love" (Jer. 31:3b).

Julie carried the burden of her abortion for several years. After the birth of her daughter, she felt the need to return to church, but she felt that she couldn't be forgiven for her abortion. She went to the pastor, who told her she could indeed be forgiven. "The reason you're hurting is because of the emotional scar, not because the sin is still there," he told her. "That was like a light bulb for me," Julie said. "That marked a turning point, and I was able to believe that I could be forgiven. I learned that I didn't need to continue to blame myself but that I was accountable only for what I had done and could be forgiven."

How does the woman receive forgiveness?

Forgiveness comes to her as a gift. God sent His Son Jesus to pay for all sins, including the abortion. Jesus died on the cross and rose again from the dead as payment for the sins of the whole world. Because Jesus died for her abortion, the woman doesn't have to be punished to pay for it. Jesus already did that for her. She only receives the gift of forgiveness by repenting of her sin and asking for God's forgiveness. When that happens, she is washed clean in God's eyes. "Though your sins are like scarlet, they shall be as white as snow; though they are red as crimson, they shall be like wool" (Isa. 1:18).

Her sin is gone; in fact, it's as if it never existed. "As far as the east is from the west, so far has he removed our transgressions from us" (Ps. 103:12). She can now live in peace here on earth and with joy that her life will continue with Christ in heaven. As a child of God, she enjoys all the blessings and love that God offers.

Forgiving others

Just as her abortion has been forgiven by God, so the woman also needs to forgive those people who were instrumental in making her abortion possible. Forgiving others is not a choice the woman has; as a forgiven sinner, she is instructed to do so. "Be kind and compassionate to one another, forgiving each other, just as in Christ God forgave you" (Eph. 4:32).

Forgiveness is relinquishing the desire to punish someone for a wrong. Just as God will not punish her for her forgiven sin, so the woman who had the abortion needs to give up her desire to punish the doctor who performed the abortion, the nurses who helped, the friend or relative who told her that she had to have the abortion, and society in general for not telling her how devastated she would feel after the abortion or for not offering alternatives to the abortion. By forgiving these people, the woman is demonstrating her gratitude for her own forgiven sin.

The woman first forgives those people in her own heart. She might even verbalize her thoughts:

"I forgive you, Mom, for not seeing my problem, for not coming to me and asking me what was wrong.

"I forgive you, Jeff, for not caring about your own unborn son or daughter, for telling me to have the abortion or you would leave me, for leaving me even after I had the abortion.

"I forgive you, Dr. Smith, and your staff, for performing the abortion. You thought you were helping me, but you only opened the doors to a life of hell. I forgive you for not telling me to have my baby, that there is help for women like me with a problem pregnancy.

"I forgive you, Alisann. You're my best friend, but you let me down when I turned to you for advice. You said abortion would solve all my problems, but it didn't. I forgive you."

Second, if possible, she should tell these same people that she forgives them. She can either tell them face-to-face or write each of them a letter expressing her forgiveness.

This will be powerful in two ways. For those people who are suffering their own guilt for aiding her in the abortion, it will relieve them to know that she does not hold them responsible. Also, if she shares with them how she has received God's forgiveness, it will be a powerful witness to them of God's love. Then they, too, can receive His forgiveness for their action or non-action and live in peace.

Maybe the people she forgives aren't even aware of what abortion really is (killing an unborn human life) or the emotional and/or physical effect it has had on her. By sharing her forgiveness with them, she will not only be educating them about the wrongness of this act but also perhaps helping to prevent future abortions. This is true especially of her doctor, who thinks he is offering a much-needed service to his patients. If he only realized the trauma abortion can cause, perhaps he would discontinue this "service." He could be the instrument to saving future unborn lives.

Confronting her doctor, friends, and family members is not an easy task. The woman shouldn't be upset with herself if this is something she cannot do. Her healing takes time and she probably won't be ready to discuss its effect on her life and how she has been forgiven until she feels at peace with herself. As she heals and becomes stronger, she can talk to them and personally offer to them the forgiveness and love that she has been carrying in her heart.

CHAPTER EIGHT

FORGIVING HERSELF

After having four abortions in five years, Deb came to know the Lord through the witness of a Christian friend. She had asked for and received God's forgiveness for her sins, especially the sin of abortion, and she thought she had forgiven herself.

As her Christian faith grew, Deb felt called to share her abortion experiences with others and soon she was speaking at pro-life meetings and sharing her story on talk shows. But as her public exposure increased, Deb began to feel uneasy about her real self—what kind of person was she to be able to kill four children? Guilt burdened her heart, reminding her of the babies who were no longer with her. She would cry because she wanted to love them so badly.

Even though she thought she had forgiven herself, Deb became confused by an unsettled feeling that wouldn't go away. "I began to think of myself as 'the woman who had four abortions' and I didn't like it." She prayed that God would take this guilt and identity from her.

God's reply came through the form of a conference on post-abortion healing, where Deb was introduced to the concept of determining the sex of her aborted babies as one step in the healing process. It sounded bizarre to her, but on her way home from the conference, she wondered if it would help her. As Deb headed out of town, the words from Psalm 27:10 spoke to her: "When mother and father forsake me, the Lord will take me up." That gave her the assurance she needed. *Yes, my children are with the Lord*, she thought. She cried softly, thinking of her four little ones, safe in heaven but so unattainable. She wanted to know more about them and she asked God to reveal to her the sex of each baby.

"I started praying and talking over all the circumstances of the first abortion. It was difficult but all these things started coming back to me that I had forgotten about. As I was talking with the Lord, I realized I was referring to the baby as 'he.' I asked God if this baby was a boy. I sensed so strongly that it was. I searched for a name and decided to name him Nathaniel."

Deb prayed over the circumstances of the other three abortions, and she sensed that another boy and then two girls that she had aborted were now with Jesus. As Deb prayed, she envisioned all four children laughing and playing at Jesus' feet. "I knew they were my babies, only they weren't so little, maybe 10, 11, 12, and 13 years old." She named the other boy Benjamin and the girls Sarah and Angelina. Then she said goodbye to them, knowing that she would see them again in heaven.

Afterward, Deb felt great relief and free from guilt. "I no longer was the woman who had four abortions, but I became the mother of four children now living in heaven with Jesus."

Many women who have had abortions, like Deb, confess their sin and ask for God's forgiveness, yet are still plagued by doubts about who they are. "How can I be a new person in Christ when I can't seem to forgive myself for what I did?"

Forgiving herself for her act of abortion is perhaps the hardest thing a woman will ever do. She can accept God's forgiveness, yet she is unable to forgive herself.

Very likely, low self-esteem was one of the factors that led to her choice of abortion. This low self-esteem is still present after the abortion. Even though she can confess her sin and accept God's forgiveness, she will have a difficult time forgiving herself. "I must be a really bad person to do something like that to my own child," she will remind herself. Her refusal to accept the freedom that forgiveness from God brings, including the freedom from self-persecution, results in unhappiness and hopelessness.

Low self-image fostered by misbeliefs

The low self-image that a woman may cling to is fostered by a number of misbeliefs that she runs through her mind like a tape-recorded message. If she ever begins to feel good about herself, she just replays one of these misbeliefs to remind herself that she is a bad person.

Some of the more common misbeliefs are:[1]

- I'm no good because of what I've done. I'm a failure at life.
- I don't deserve any happiness.
- I must always pay for the bad things that I do.
- I will never get over my abortion; I'm stuck with this pain and guilt the rest of my life.
- What others think is vitally important to my happiness.
- I have to be perfect; I can't let anyone know what I did.

---

[1]William Backus, Ph.D., *Telling the Truth to Troubled People*, Fourth National Lutherans For Life Convention, November 2, 1985, Minneapolis, MN, workshop notes.

By holding on to the misbeliefs, the woman is preventing true healing to occur and will not be at peace with herself.

For three and a half years of marriage, Sarah hid the secret of her past abortion from her husband and attempted to bury her feelings of being a bad person. Two doctors and her pastor had advised Sarah not to tell her husband about her affair with a married man that had ended in abortion.

When her husband wanted to start a family, all the guilt and unhappy memories of her abortion confronted her. She also felt dishonest for marrying her husband when he believed her to be a pure, chaste woman.

Desperately needing to talk to someone about her situation, Sarah contacted a local minister, who suggested she follow the guidelines listed in a paper entitled "The Healing Steps":[2]

1. *Relax.* "Be still, and know that I am God" (Ps. 46:10). In seeking the healing grace of God, the woman's body must be free of all tension so that her mind can concentrate on God's mercy and love.

2. *Cleanse.* "If we walk in the light as he is in the light, we have fellowship with one another and the blood of Jesus, his Son, purifies us from all sin" (1 John 1:7). The woman must confess her sins without reserve, and never explain or excuse them. Also, she must refuse to keep a secret hold on her sins after she has confessed to God and received His forgiveness.

3. *Clarify.* "Jesus stopped and called to them: 'What do you want me to do for you?' " (Matt. 20:32). The woman seeking healing must not be vague. She must tell God the specific area in which she needs healing, such as forgiving herself.

---

[2]Sarah Williams, "Even in the Wilderness, Forgiveness Lives," *Focus on the Family* (July 1987), p. 7.

4. *Consecrate.* "Whether we live or die, we belong to the Lord" (Rom. 14:8). One of the conditions of divine healing is the spiritual attitude that the woman totally relinquishes her life to the will of God.

5. *Anticipate.* "Faith is the substance of things hoped for, the evidence of things not seen" (Heb. 11:1). She should always anticipate God fulfilling what He has already promised to do.

6. *Appropriate.* "I can do all things through Christ who gives me strength" (Phil. 4:13). The woman receives what God has promised, acts in the strength of the healing power received, and is grateful to God for the salvation He offers to her.

Sarah followed these steps daily for several months, and continued to pray for guidance. As her relationship with the Lord blossomed, she spent several days alone, when she fasted and prayed. "I could never deny or forget what had been, but it didn't have to dictate my todays. I retraced the painful experiences of my past with God and bathed in His forgiveness. Finally, I was able to forgive myself." She later told her husband about her abortion and he, too, forgave her.

Why does the woman need to forgive herself?

The woman who does not forgive herself will be burdened with a guilt that, if left unexamined, will demand repayment in one of two ways: in the form of false justification or by turning in on oneself.[3]

With false justification, the woman will continue to become pregnant and have abortions to justify that what she did with the first pregnancy was the right thing to do. By repeatedly turning to abortion as the answer, she rein-

---

[3]James Wheeler, S.J., "The Quality of Mercy: Healing Prayer in Abortion's Aftermath," *Journal of Christian Healing* (Vol. 7, No. 2), p. 41.

forces that she did the right thing in the first place. The more abortions she has, the easier it becomes to have them, and to justify having them.

Sandi had blocked the details of her three abortions, and until she became a Christian, didn't see anything wrong with abortion. "Before I was saved, I never felt that abortion was wrong or had any guilt. I viewed being pregnant as an inconvenience and didn't want to be bothered with it. Abortion just didn't cross my mind as something I needed to be sorry about."

To rationalize her abortions, Sandi convinced herself that she hated children and never wanted to be a mother. Eventually, she had a tubal ligation so that she would never become pregnant again.

But after she became a Christian, Sandi's heart softened and she realized that her hatred toward children was an emotional effect of her abortions. "The Lord began showing me how I had been affected by the abortions, and I realized that I was a sinner. I knew I had to truly repent of my abortions because the Lord wanted me to. I got into the Word of God and read books and studied. There have been times of true inner searching and weeping but not a depressed weeping. I have felt a cleansing within myself as I continue to receive God's forgiveness and love."

If a woman hasn't forgiven herself for the abortion, she may turn the guilt in on herself. When this happens, she will see only the wrongness of what she did and will not be able to live with the self-hatred. Ultimately, she will contemplate committing suicide and may even make an attempt on her own life. For her own protection, she needs to confront her abortion before her life loses all meaning and she decides to end it.

In Deb's situation, her guilt over her four abortions tormented her daily. When she wasn't working, she would stay in bed and think about the babies she had killed. She became interested in the occult and astrology, spending hours charting her future. After she suspected she was pregnant for the fifth time, this time as the result of an extramarital affair, Deb really dwelled on her abortions and vowed to never have another one. But the guilt dragged her down and her future looked hopeless. Her marriage was falling apart and she expected her husband to leave her soon for another woman.

One cold January night, as Deb folded laundry in her basement she reflected on the downward spiral of her life. She felt a tremendous desire to end it all. She found her husband's shotgun and then stood over him as he lay asleep on the living room couch. "I hate you, I hate you," she repeated aloud, intent on killing herself before him.

Before Deb pulled the trigger, she heard a loud whooshing noise in the basement. Snapped out of her trance, Deb ran downstairs to find that the hoses had come loose from the washing machine. Water sprayed across the room, soaking stacked boxes, walls, ceiling, as well as the clean clothes piled on top of the dryer. The mess distracted her from her suicide attempt. Within days, her Christian friend at work began talking to Deb. As a result, Deb placed the pieces of her life into the hands of Jesus.

Sorting out the blame

A woman who has chosen abortion needs to reconcile with herself, to sort out the blame for what happened. She needs to ask herself, "What am I responsible for and what are others responsible for?" To do this, she needs to reflect on what happened in her life from the moment she suspected or learned that she was pregnant. The following questions might help her remember the thoughts and events that led to her abortion:

• What were my initial feelings? Was I excited at

first, only to have reality set in and tell me I couldn't possibly have a baby?
- Why was it so impossible not to carry my baby to term? Was it because I was unmarried, in school, or not financially ready for a baby? Was I just picking up on a career that I had let go to raise my first three children?
- Did I feel unstable and unable to handle the pressure of raising a child alone?

Whatever her reasons, it might be helpful if the woman could actually list them on paper, then examine each one and evaluate its validity. After considering the circumstances surrounding her abortion, she should try to remember the people who influenced her decision to have the abortion by asking herself these questions:

- Did they tell me abortion was my only option?
- Did my parents threaten to disown me if I didn't have the abortion?
- Did the father of the baby promise to leave me if I had the baby?
- Just how much of the decision to abort was mine and how much did other people influence me?

Besides circumstances and people who might have influenced the woman to abort, she needs to reflect on her spiritual life at the time of the abortion. Was she a Christian when she had the abortion? The following verse might help her to understand why she chose abortion even as a Christian: "These people come near to me with their mouth and honor me with their lips, but their hearts are far from me. Their worship of me is made up only of rules taught by men" (Isa. 29:13).

Perhaps she was attending church at the time, but she really didn't have a personal relationship with the Lord.

She knew He existed and recognized His power and ability, but maybe she had never gone to Him with her own personal problems and needs. The distance between her and God may have been too great to ever approach Him or go to Him for help. She would have had more of an intellectual knowledge of God rather than a personal relationship with a Father who wants to take care of His child.

After answering the questions relating to the circumstances leading to her abortion and people who influenced her, as well as considering her spiritual life, the woman should understand her role and admit her responsibility for her part in the abortion. Other people and the circumstances may have influenced her decision, but she still had a part in that decision.

Sinners are lovable

Despite her responsibility for her abortion, the woman needs to believe in her heart that she is lovable, that she has self-worth. She needs to understand what it means to truly love herself: to see herself as a gift that God has created. For this to happen, she must feel the touch of Jesus' love.

Jesus' love and self-forgiveness go hand-in-hand. With His love, the woman hurt by abortion can make changes in her life; she can discard her old self-image and take on a new one. With the courage of love, she can dare to forgive herself.[4]

Before she knew about Jesus' forgiveness for her, Karen was an independent, hardened young woman who had lived on her own since the age of 15. She had run away

---

[4]Lewis B. Smedes, *Forgive and Forget: Putting the Past Behind You*, pamphlet produced by Focus on the Family, P.O. Box 500, Arcadia, CA 91006 (copyright 1987), p. 4.

from her alcoholic father and their fights. Over the next seven years, she became pregnant four times, giving the first baby up for adoption and aborting the other three. Karen lived a promiscuous lifestyle, perpetuating her hatred of men.

But a Christian man won her heart and after their marriage, Karen came to know Jesus as her Savior. As a Christian, she recognized that her three abortions were sins for which she needed to repent. She also realized that her abortions had fostered a growing self-hatred that had led to her promiscuous lifestyle. As a born-again Christian, Karen studied the Bible, hungry for the words that described Jesus' love for her.

Today, Karen still has the strength and boldness of her teen years, but now she finds her strength in the Holy Spirit. "My goal is to make Satan regret he ever made sin look good to me. I want him to tremble." As an active pro-life leader, Karen speaks publicly about her abortion experiences and their effects on her. "I want other women to understand how abortion can affect their lives and, despite what they've done, that they are lovable in God's eyes."

God forgives abortion

A woman who has had an abortion needs to know that God forgives her sins through Jesus Christ, who suffered on the cross, died, and rose again. All she has to do is believe that Jesus is the one who can save her. Because of what He did, she does not have to be punished for her sins if she confesses that she did sin and is sorry for them.

Her guilt can lead her in one of two directions: If she is unrepentant, she is condemned to spend eternity in hell, but if she confesses her sins and believes that Jesus has suffered for her, then she is convinced that she is saved. It's like being locked in a cell with her sins, with no means of escape. Then God gives her the key (Jesus) to open the door and be set free.

As a forgiven sinner, the woman can claim the promise that God offers in the Bible:

"Therefore, there is now no condemnation for those who are in Christ Jesus, because through Christ Jesus the law of the Spirit of Life set me free from the law of sin and death" (Rom. 8:1–2).

All the woman needs to do is accept the gift of God's healing. Faith is the basis for accepting this gift and is made up of two parts: God's belief in the woman and her belief in God.

The woman must decide to forgive herself

Forgiving herself is a decision that the woman must make on her own. But, at the same time, she needs to recognize that the power to forgive herself and turn her life around is found in Christ. James 4:10 says, "Humble yourselves before the Lord and he will lift you up."

If she continues to fear God's punishment and to punish herself, the woman is denying the power of Christ's death to cleanse her of her sins and she is doubting God's love for her.

If you've had an abortion

It is possible for you to forgive yourself. You do not have to live with your self-hatred the rest of your life. To reach this point in your healing, you might find the following suggestions helpful:

1. The most powerful tool you have is prayer. At any time, you can turn to God and pray, especially for the healing of the memory of the abortion and for release from

guilt. You can also pray that God will enable you to see yourself as He sees you and to forgive yourself. Thank God that you recognize that your sorrow over your sin has brought you to repentance and everlasting life. "Godly sorrow brings repentance that leads to salvation and leaves no regret, but worldly sorrow brings death. See what this godly sorrow has produced in you: what earnestness, what eagerness to clear yourselves, what indignation, what alarm, what longing, what concern, what readiness to see justice done" (2 Cor. 7:10–11).

Mona felt burdened with the guilt of her abortion, even though she knew God forgave her for her sin. She felt that she would be punished and lived in fear. Her only relief came when she took her fear and guilt to God. "I know what I did was wrong and it's frustrating for me knowing that I killed the only child I will probably ever have with my husband. But when I turned my fear and guilt over to God through constant prayer, I was able to accept what happened. I still struggle with the guilt, and I pray daily that it, too, will leave me."

2. (Publisher's note: We recognize that communion, as a sacrament, is not observed universally in the church. It is important, however, to acknowledge the significance it holds for believers of many denominations.) If you are a member of a Christian church, you can celebrate the Sacrament of Holy Communion either during a communion service with other members of your church or privately with your pastor or priest. To prepare for partaking of the sacrament you should ask yourself, how do I perceive God's feelings about me at this moment? What spiritual healing or gift do I pray for through this sacrament? As you celebrate the sacrament, visualize a loving and healing God who wants to cleanse you of all guilt and self-hatred. Michael Mannion, who has counseled hundreds of women post-abortion through his campus ministry, be-

lieves that the Sacrament of Holy Communion is a means for the woman to receive God's mercy. "The role of the priest in the Sacrament is to definitively proclaim God's healing to a sister in Christ. The priest is no better than she, for he, too, is a sinner. In fact, it is God's irony and choice that he uses the broken to announce his wholeness, the fellow sinner to announce the presence of He who was without sin (Jesus)."[5]

3. A caring network of other women who have suffered from the emotional effects of abortion and have been healed will be an invaluable support. You can restore your life with the help of a loving Christian community. Local support groups can be found in the telephone directory under abortion counseling or crisis pregnancy centers. (Appendix C lists specific support groups that might be available in your area.)

One of the first post-abortion support groups, Women Exploited By Abortion (WEBA), was founded by Nancyjo Mann, who had an abortion in her fifth month of pregnancy. After sharing the effects of her abortion, other women deluged her with letters and phone calls. They too had been suffering from Post Abortion Syndrome but didn't realize it. By sharing their experiences with each other, these women formed a support network that promoted emotional and spiritual healing. From one woman and her abortion testimony, WEBA has grown to more than 15,000 members, all of whom have suffered from the emotional effects of abortion.

4. If you feel comfortable expressing your feelings on paper, you can write a poem or song to your aborted baby or to God. Nancyjo Mann composed the following poem, which can be sung to the tune of "Brahm's Lullaby," as a

---

[5]Father Michael T. Mannion, S.T.L., M.A., *Abortion & Healing: A Cry to Be Whole* (Kansas City, Mo.: Sheed and Ward, 1986), p. 88.

way of expressing her love for the little girl she aborted:

> My Shauna Marie, it's been several years,
>   since I cried my very first tear.
> The years have gone by and though I have tried,
>   I've never ever forgotten you, dear.
> I'd hold deep inside my feelings I hide,
>   and yet they never would go.
> So I brought into light my heartache to sight
>   and admitted that now, now it must go.

By writing down your feelings, you can deal with them more honestly and they become more valid.

5. You can commit the baby to God. The process of letting your baby come to life in your mind (which is not the same as "New Age" visualization) so that you can know that it was real and then allowing it to die so that you can grieve was described in detail in Chapter Four. Not only should you let the baby die, but you should commit the baby to God's care, so that you can find comfort knowing that your child is in a wonderful haven, free from pain or sin. Do this alone or with the help of a Christian counselor, who will lead you through the imaging of the baby being presented to God.

Connie realized that she needed professional counseling about two years after her abortion. She had been burdened by the guilt over what she had done and thought about her abortion every day. When she wasn't working at her job as a librarian, she would curl up on her sofa and think about the baby she had killed. She had no desire to go out with her friends and rarely called her family, who didn't know about the abortion. Connie had been a member of a local church for many years, but had a difficult time sitting through church services. She would start to cry whenever the pastor talked about God's forgiveness, because she felt she couldn't be forgiven.

"I desperately wanted God to help me, but I felt so unlovable. Finally, I went to my pastor and confessed my abortion, asking him how I could let go of my baby and get on with my life. He began counseling me and explained that I needed to break the spiritual bond I had with my baby. I had to let God take care of my baby."

Through weekly prayer sessions, Connie gradually let go of her baby. First, she let the baby be real in her mind by deciding that the baby was a girl. She named her Heather and spoke to God about what type of person Heather was: a loving, happy little girl who knew and loved Jesus.

Then, with her pastor's help, she let the baby die by recalling the abortion itself and what happened during the procedure. She remembered the pain and the repulsion she felt when she saw the tube connected to the suction machine fill with red blood and pieces of her baby. Feeling cold and empty, Connie wept uncontrollably for Heather.

But instead of leaving the baby's pieces in the suction machine, Connie envisioned a whole Heather, wrapped in a pink blanket, being presented to Jesus to care for. As Connie placed her daughter in Jesus' arms, Heather smiled at her with her tiny rosebud lips. "I commit my child to you, Lord," Connie prayed, feeling a deep sense of relief and peace. She now knew that Heather was in heaven and would know no more pain. Connie was able to get on with her own life.

Healing is a process, not an event. You need to recognize that you will not be healed overnight, but that the healing will develop in stages. With God's help, you will find true peace and meaning to your abortion in the right time.

CHAPTER NINE

LIVING WITH A FORGIVEN ABORTION

In Chapter Five we told Robin's story. Eighteen years old, she did not want to marry the father of her baby or give the child up for adoption. Her search for an unwed mothers' home in which to have her baby ended when her doctor and a social worker encouraged her to have an abortion.

Since abortion was not yet legal, two psychiatrists were asked to certify the necessity of abortion for emotional reasons. "One of the psychiatrists asked me a few questions and then said I was crazy, which justified the abortion," Robin said. "I believed him."

Afterward, Robin moved to get away from the nightmare she had suffered. "I wanted to forget the whole thing, but it was always there," she said. "Every day it haunted me, whispering in my ear, 'Abortion, abortion, you're awful.'"

Eventually she married and bore two children, but Robin couldn't forget her abortion. The guilt hung over her like a cloud. She avoided conversation and rarely talked about her abortion. Only her husband and a few friends knew about her experience. "Finally I said to myself, 'I'm going crazy; I've got to do something.' So I went to a therapist who happened to be a Christian and he shared the forgiveness that was available for me through Jesus Christ. I accepted Jesus into my life and knew that I was forgiven for my abortion."

With additional counseling and Bible study, Robin began the healing process, and within three years, she forgave herself for having the abortion. She decided to contact WEBA (Woman Exploited By Abortion) to see if she could help them.

"After I heard a speaker tell about her abortion experience, I knew that's what the Lord wanted me to do. I had been so shy before but He enables me to share my story." Robin now travels to national leadership conferences and to local and statewide meetings to talk about her abortion and, hopefully, reach other women who have suffered the emotional effects of an abortion. Currently she serves as the regional director for Open Arms, a national post-abortion healing group. With God's forgiveness and direction, she has turned a bad experience into a meaningful ministry.

When is a woman healed?

The woman who has had an abortion enters the final stages of healing when she takes her eyes off her pain and seeks the Lord and His plan for her life. She wants His direction and asks for it. "For I know the plans I have for you," declares the Lord, "plans to prosper you and not to harm you, plans to give you hope and a future. Then you will call upon me and come and pray to me, and I will listen to you" (Jer. 29:11–12).

To help her know that healing has or is taking place,

the woman might find it helpful to answer the following questions:[1]

1. Has she returned to her previous level of functioning? Is she actively involved in daily living and interested in what is going on around her?

If she was a student at the time of her abortion, she should be continuing her studies and making plans for her life after graduation. If a wife and mother, she should be involved in her family's activities and fulfilling her role expectations. If actively pursuing a career, she should once again be busy with her job, functioning as she did prior to the abortion. Her goals may be different and she may have grown emotionally and spiritually from her abortion experience, but she will not separate herself from the living world.

2. Has she set aside the defenses of denial?

Healing is taking place when the woman no longer rationalizes her abortion. She will readily admit that she made a wrong choice and will know that she has been forgiven for her abortion.

3. Has she experienced the child as being real and mourned the loss appropriately?

As part of her healing, she will know that she aborted a human life, her child, and not just a blob of tissue. The aborted fetus becomes "her baby" and her baby has been killed. She will grieve for the loss of her child and recognize that he or she was a real part of her life, if only for a short while.

4. Can she imagine the baby at peace with God?

With healing, the woman will not grieve indefinitely. As with all losses, she will come to terms with the death of her child and understand that the baby is now in

---

[1]Dr. E. Joanne Angelo, "The Healing Process," presented at Healing Visions, the First National Conference on Post Abortion Counseling, University of Notre Dame (August 12, 1986).

heaven, where there is no pain or sorrow.

5. Does she believe God forgives her?

The woman who is healed will believe that God forgives her for her abortion. She will have confessed her sin and asked for forgiveness. She will accept His forgiveness and believe that she is without sin in His sight, through the saving grace of Jesus' death and resurrection. She has turned away from the belief that she can never be absolved for what she has done.

6. Has she forgiven herself?

A woman will not only have accepted God's forgiveness, but she will have forgiven herself for her abortion. The little voice won't whisper in her ear, "Murderer, murderer!" She won't avoid interacting with people at work or church for fear of what they would think if they found out she had an abortion. Her abortion won't be a controlling part of her anymore, because it has been forgiven. Instead of the woman who had an abortion, she will think of herself as a child of God, precious to Him and full of worth. She is somebody!

7. Has she found meaning in the tragedy?

The woman will have processed the abortion experience in the context of her whole life. She will have considered how it happened, why it happened, and what she has learned from the experience. By gaining insight into why she made the abortion decision, she will have an understanding of her own weaknesses and needs.

If you've had an abortion

If you are still healing emotionally from your abortion and need some extra guidance to put your experience behind you, you might find it helpful to set goals to give you guidelines for daily living. The following goals were compiled by members of a post-abortion mutual support group:[2]

1. To be able to verbalize my feelings and emotions.

You should strive to put into words how you feel about your abortion and its effect on you. In the process, you won't feel "empty inside" anymore. You will also respond to tragedies and sad events, instead of feeling nothing. Allow yourself to be happy again and laugh so you can react to the world around you and not hide.

2. To be able to handle fear of what others might say when they hear of my abortion.

If a friend or acquaintance asks you about your abortion, be ready to respond with an honest reply. Don't be afraid of what that person must think of you. Rather, have the self-confidence to admit that you made a mistake and that you have learned from it. You may even share what effect the abortion has had on your life and how you have grown from it.

3. To be sensitive and open to God as to when to share my experience and not to share it indiscriminately.

Do not feel compelled to tell everyone about your experience. Rather, through daily prayer and an open relationship with God, you will know when to talk about your abortion. It won't be a burden for the rest of your life; it will become a tool that God uses to reach other hurting women.

4. To understand how the abortion has changed my decision-making process in order to help or warn others.

You will have analyzed why and how your abortion took place, based on the thought process you used at the time. You will have learned where you were vulnerable and at what point you shut out the medical facts. You will

---

[2]Handout from Save-a-Life, Ramsay Building, Suite 112, 1608 13th Avenue South, Birmingham, AL 35205 (February 1986).

understand your weaknesses in handling a crisis and what you based your abortion decision on. With this self-analysis, you will have a clear understanding of how your abortion came to be. You will recognize this same process in other women who may be considering abortion and be able to counsel them. Your advice will have greater impact on their final abortion decision because you've been there and speak from experience.

5. To react properly to children (not to coddle excessively, reject, or expect too much of them).

Attempt to respond to children in a loving manner, not thinking of them as replacements for your lost child but as individuals who deserve your respect. Do not be overly protective or totally reject them and their needs. Rather, allow them to grow as individuals and don't attempt to mold them into the person you wanted your aborted child to be.

6. To learn the proper ways of handling anger.

Do not turn your anger outward toward others in your life or inward toward yourself. Rather, consider why you are angry. Does it relate to your abortion experience? Are you still blaming someone else or something else for your abortion? Anger in itself is not bad if it serves as an outlet for unexpressed emotions. But you should attempt to understand what emotions lie behind the anger. Are you still suffering from unresolved grief that you have denied? By stepping back and considering what made you angry, you will gain a better understanding of your own emotions.

7. To learn how to forgive myself.

Whenever doubts about your self-worth arise, you may want to read Scripture verses dealing with forgiveness (see Appendix A) or pray about your feelings. Also, you can become active in women's Bible studies, join a post-abortion support group, and work at a project that you excel in. If you are a full-time mother and housewife, you might want to perform a service for your loved ones, such as organizing a family outing or preparing a special meal. Or you could volunteer for an assignment at work that you would enjoy and accomplish well.

What you are attempting to do through these various activities is to remind yourself that you do have value and your life does have meaning. As a forgiven person, you have left behind your old choices and way of life and are a new creature in God's eyes. Don't dwell on your past, but use it to minister to other hurting people.

8. To learn how to be vulnerable in front of others.

Whenever confronted with a situation where you feel as if you are exposing your most tender emotions, allow yourself to openly express those feelings. Don't hold back tears of sadness or joy. Experience your emotions without feeling the need to explain them.

9. To be happy with myself.

Whenever you catch yourself pointing out your own weakness, complaining that you're not "bright enough" or "pretty enough," remember that you were created by God and are special in His sight. You have unique qualities unlike any other person and, as a child of God, you have the most important gift: eternal life.

10. To trust men more.

You might want to ask a male friend you feel comfortable with to help you in this area. Tell him the difficulty you have trusting men in general and ask him to be your friend, to teach you how males think and why they react differently than women to life's crises. Perhaps he could help you understand why the male doctor or your father recommended the abortion without seeming to be bothered by your emotions or needs.

The male friend you confide in could be a co-worker, a neighbor, or someone from your church. He might even be a boyfriend or husband. As you begin to trust him more, consciously work at developing relationships with other males in your life. Don't avoid interacting with someone because of his gender.

11. To handle feelings of being exploited.

If you decide to publicly share your abortion experience, there may be times when you feel used by pro-life groups or your church as they put you in a position where you relate your abortion story. You may feel as if people ask you to share your experience only because it will attract people to a meeting or seminar and not because you want to discourage other people from making the same mistake. You might think, "Nobody cared about me before they knew I had an abortion, but now I'm known as the woman who aborted her baby."

If you truly believe that you are being exploited, then step back from the public light and examine why you want to share your story. Perhaps your feeling of being used is really a reflection of your own need to justify your abortion. If you don't feel the need to share your experience, then you should talk to the people who are encouraging your public testimony and ask them to limit your exposure.

These 11 goals are designed to help you rebuild your self-esteem and self-confidence. Because you normally acquire your sense of self-worth from your immediate family, you should work to resolve any family conflicts. Spend time nearly every day becoming more intimate with your mate and children. Parents, brothers, sisters, and other close relatives should also have a high priority. The intimacy you enjoy with your family is more vital to your mental health than you can imagine.

Free from guilt

A woman can be assured that she is indeed free from the bond of guilt and should have a clear conscience. "Let us draw near to God with a sincere heart in full assurance of faith, having our hearts sprinkled to cleanse us from a guilty conscience and having our bodies washed with pure water" (Heb. 10:22).

Because she is free from the bond of guilt, the woman can live a life that glorifies God. No longer does the weight of her guilt drag her down, like an iron ball chained to her leg. She has been released of her burden. As a forgiven person, she can let her Christian life be an example for other people, so that they, too, can turn to God for forgiveness and eternal life. She also will glorify God by loving all people (no matter what their color or nationality or physical ability), forgiving all who might hurt her, and actively sharing the message of Jesus' forgiveness.

Jennifer, whose story opened this book, has gone from a state of suicidal depression over her abortion to living a life that glorifies God. After publicly committing her life to Christ, she became active in pro-life groups and women's post-abortion support groups. She is now a director for Open Arms, a post-abortion group, for which she counsels women suffering from PAS and gives public testimony of her own abortion experience. She is married to a Christian and is raising her daughter and son to know the Lord.

Because she has been freed from her abortion guilt, the woman is free to forgive herself and to forgive others. In fact, as a Christian, she is instructed to put forgiveness into action. "We love because he first loved us. If anyone says, 'I love God,' yet hates his brother, he is a liar. For anyone who does not love his brother, whom he has seen, cannot love God, whom he has not seen" (1 John 4:19–20).

So if a woman has truly been forgiven for her abortion, she will in turn forgive others for their sins against her. Her forgiveness will not be passive; rather, she will put her forgiveness into action and clear up any wrongs that resulted from her abortion.

After Deb accepted Jesus' forgiveness for her four abortions, she realized that she needed to pay back the money she had stolen to pay for her first abortion. She went to the bank where she had worked at the time and explained to her former supervisor that she had stolen some money and wanted to return it. "I told her that Jesus had come into my life and I realized I needed to repay the money I had stolen," Deb said. The woman was shocked, but impressed, with Deb's honesty and faith.

Listening to God

The woman needs to be receptive to God's direction in her life, to listen to His plans for her. She does this by a regular prayer life, where she talks to God, asking for His guidance and peace, and then waiting for Him to respond. She also reads the Bible, aware that God speaks to her through Scripture. If she feels called to publicly share her story in order to help other women become healed, then she needs to feel God's peace that it is His will that she do this.

To what ministry does God call her?

Is it the ministry of reconciliation, where she can be an instrument in bringing other women to receive God's forgiveness and be reconciled to His love? This could be done by personally telling her story on an individual basis with women who call and talk to her about their own abortions. Perhaps they saw her story in the newspaper or church magazine and want to learn more about how they, too, can be forgiven.

Jane now shares her two abortion experiences publicly

and with individuals, with the purpose of showing how God's love turned her life from despair to joy. She serves as a WEBA counselor, so her telephone number is available to women who might need someone to talk to about their own abortion experience. "I want to tell people about all the love that Jesus has for them. If they don't accept it, they are missing out. He wants to give so much, and all we have to do is accept Him. I get so excited thinking how, before I accepted Jesus, my life was nowhere and now it's somewhere: in heaven!"

Is the woman called to the ministry of counseling those who are suffering from the anguish of their own abortion to offer comfort and steps to healing? If so, she might serve as a counselor for a crisis pregnancy center telephone hotline or lead support group sessions for women suffering from PAS. She may even be led to seek a counseling degree so that she can work full time as a professional counselor.

Janna, who had an abortion during the 16th week of her pregnancy, works one hour every day as a telephone counselor for Conquerors, a post-abortion support group in Minnesota. In addition, she leads weekly group sessions where the women are taken through the steps of post-abortion healing. "I see my counseling other women as a natural step from my own healing," Janna said. "I want to help them the way I've been helped."

Or is the woman called to use her abortion experience to glorify the Lord as Paul did in Acts 26:29? "Paul replied, 'Short time or long—I pray God that not only you but all who are listening to me today may become what I am, except for these chains.' " Paul is referring to his conversion from one who persecuted Christians to a sinner who came to know Jesus and trust in Him as his Savior. Many people came to know of Jesus' saving love because they wanted to know how a cruel person such as Paul could change so suddenly and so drastically. Likewise, the woman who is healed through Jesus can be a great witness to those around her. For some, friends will notice the difference from her previous way of life. She can witness her experience, whether publicly or privately, to the glory of God.

And finally, her personal experience with abortion and subsequent knowledge of the abortion procedure may lead the woman to a ministry of working to end the legalization of abortion in the United States or to discourage people from accepting it as a logical and harmless procedure. She knows what abortion does, both to the developing baby and to the mother, and she may choose to actively work toward exposing the truth about abortion.

Called according to talents

Each woman's ministry will be unique because each will be called according to her own talents. However, all will be serving the same purpose by the same Spirit. "There are different kinds of gifts, but the same Spirit. There are different kinds of service, but the same Lord. There are different kinds of working, but the same God works all of them in all men" (1 Cor. 12:4).

The woman who didn't know Christ before her abortion will want to serve God and look to Him for direction. "Therefore, prepare your minds for action; be self-controlled; set your hope fully on the grace to be given you when Jesus Christ is revealed. As obedient children, do not conform to the evil desires you had when you lived in ignorance. But just as he who called you is holy, so be holy in all you do; for it is written: 'Be holy, because I am holy' " (1 Pet. 1:13–16).

A woman is ready to make a commitment to the pro-life ministry when she comes forward not out of guilt but from freewill and healed conviction.

If you've had an abortion

Before you commit your life to an active ministry, whether it's working for a pro-life group or serving as a volunteer for a post-abortion support group, first examine your motive. Ask yourself: Am I doing this out of love for others and thankfulness for my own healing, or will it help justify my own abortion?

If you feel truly grateful for having been emotionally healed of your abortion and desire to help other women find that same peace, then you can be confident that your motive is healthy.

Before deciding the area of ministry on which you wish to focus time and energy, first ask God to direct you in your efforts. Pray that He gives you peace of mind about your chosen field and that He blesses your work. And as you strive to help others, may your prayer be as joyful as the post-aborted woman who expressed her feelings in the following verse:

"So many small lives taken,
Too many women aching!
Thank you, Jesus, for being alive,
I'm forgiven of my crime!"

CHAPTER TEN

ABORTION AFFECTS FATHERS, CHILDREN

The abortion of his firstborn has left 48-year-old James angry.

"There's lots of anger in guys," James said. "The ones blowing up clinics are guys. They don't have control. They can't legislate and say this is my body and my baby and I'm going to keep it. They have to try to convince the girl that that's my son or daughter in there; I don't want you to destroy it. Basically, the guy can't do anything; he has to sit back and watch."

James rarely tells people about his abortion experience, but agreed to share it with the author so that others will realize that fathers of aborted babies can be devastated by the procedure.

James and Kathy had been married one year when Kathy became pregnant with their first child. James didn't feel very enthusiastic about the pregnancy. "I felt kind of strange and not ready to start a family. I let her decide what she wanted to do," he said. "She wasn't ready for a family either."

Kathy suggested that she have an abortion. James didn't have any strong feelings about it either way. "I didn't think about it. I never even thought about what it meant. It wasn't a big thing back in those days." So he went along with her decision to abort the 12-week-old fetus.

After the couple arrived at the clinic for the procedure, James began to feel ambivalent about what they were doing. "Abortion wasn't widely publicized [at that time], but there was something bad about it that bothered me."

In the clinic parking lot, James noticed all the men waiting there, pacing or talking to each other. Some smoked cigarettes; others smoked grass or were drinking.

"I sat in the car for a while after Kathy went in, but then I got out and talked to the other guys. A lot of them were ambivalent about abortion. It was really strange but a lot of them didn't really want it. It was like they were doing it for their girlfriends or their wives. That's when I felt like I wanted to go inside and stop the whole thing. It just hit me, good grief, this is a baby. But even if I had gotten in there, I wouldn't have known which way to go or where to find them or anything. I've often thought about how I could have tried to stop it."

Later, James found out that Kathy had wanted to stop the abortion after she was in the clinic. She had cried and wanted to tell the people to stop, but once the procedure started, she felt she had to go through with it.

"She wanted to say no," said James, "and I wanted to run in, but neither of us knew it. If she had come out still pregnant, I would have been happy."

After a couple hours, Kathy did come out, but with a different look in her eyes. "We rode quietly and went straight back to Chicago. It was a traumatic experience. We knew we had done wrong when we were leaving the place. It was quiet. No words were spoken. Later on Kathy cried about it and we talked. She said something about how she could feel this pulling or tugging inside of her.

All I could imagine was the baby trying to hang on to her insides as the doctor was pulling him out. He was just a teeny weeny little guy.''

Four years later, James and Kathy became Christians and at that time they prayed for forgiveness for their abortion as they wept for the baby who had no way of coming back into their lives.

About a year later, James dreamt that he died and went to heaven, where he was met at the gates by a little boy. "Right away, I knew who he was. I walked right up to him and said, 'You're my first son and your name is Joel.' He put his arms around me and held me. Then someone appeared and said to me, 'You know, you had two choices. You could have either rejected or ignored this little fellow standing here or you could have embraced him as your own son. He truly is your son and he is a fine boy. But he didn't have a name and he wanted to know what you wanted to call him.' I was really nuts about him, but I had to wake up. He's 15 years old now. All night long I was crying and the next day I was thinking about that dream. I still dream about Joel every once in while."

Little has been written about fathers of aborted babies: how they feel about the abortion, the effects of the abortion on their lives, and how abortion has changed their lives. Legally, fathers have no rights to prevent abortion and need not be informed that an abortion is to be performed on their offspring. How much the fathers get involved often depends on the mothers.

Those fathers who know about the pregnancy and participate in the abortion decision may be very supportive and even accompany the woman to the abortion clinic. Others, especially those who strongly oppose the abortion, will not have anything to do with arranging the abortion or going to the clinic with the woman. Some men who oppose the abortion may still feel a responsibility in helping the woman secure or pay for the abortion and may accompany her to the clinic. Still others are ignorant that the woman is even pregnant and are never told that their child was aborted. Each of these categories of fathers reacts differently to the abortion experience, but all will share some common effects.

Sociologist Arthur Shostak, a professor at Drexel University in Philadelphia and father of an aborted child, has spent more than ten years studying the impact of abortion on men. Although a pro-choice advocate, he has concluded that abortion is a great, unrecognized trauma for males, perhaps the only major trauma that most men go through without seeking professional counseling.[1] Shostak, with writer Gary McLouth, surveyed 1,000 males in 18 states who had accompanied the mother of their child to abortion clinics. The results, discussed in their book *Men and Abortion: Lessons, Losses, and Love*, showed that most of the men felt isolation, anger, and fear of the emotional and physical damage to the women. While the purpose of accompanying the woman to the clinic was to support and console her, 88% of the clinics who participated in the research barred men from the procedure and the recovery room.[2] This left the men alone in the waiting room, with their concerns and frustrations.

Role confusion

Men are expected to be strong, aggressive, and responsible. The phrase "act like a man" brings to mind a muscular, powerful aggressor who will stop at nothing to protect his rights. Even the male sex role has been categorized by researchers and therapists according to the typical male attributes: dominancy/power, aggression/activity,

---

[1]John Leo, "Sharing the Pain of Abortion," *Time* (September 26, 1983), p. 78.
[2]Ibid., p. 78.

self-reliance/autonomy, achievement/success, and responsibility/protectiveness. But an abortion experience contradicts the expected male sex role in each of these areas.[3]

Dominancy/power

While women have gained new levels of freedom and power in the work force, our society is still male dominated, except in the area of abortion, where women maintain absolute control. Despite his opinions, beliefs, personal feelings, or desire to financially support the child, the male has no legal or personal rights in the issue of abortion. Thus, the abortion experience leaves him with the sense of utter powerlessness and frustration.

Also, if the father does not know about the abortion, he may experience frustration over a relationship that suddenly changes, for no apparent reason.

Richard sought marital counseling when he felt his wife rejecting him but he couldn't understand why. Through separate interviews with the couple, the counselor learned that the wife had an affair several years earlier which resulted in a pregnancy by her lover. She had an abortion and didn't tell her husband about the pregnancy or the abortion. The hostility Richard had been experiencing was the result of his wife's fear of admitting her extramarital affair. As a result, she would not let him get close to her or love her and he didn't understand why.

Aggression/Activity

Where man is expected to be in control of his life and to be able to change his environment, he finds with abortion that he has no ability to change anything. His role is

---

[3]Dr. Vincent M. Rue, "Abortion in Relationship Context," *International Review of Natural Family Planning* (Summer 1985), pp. 100–104.

usually passive and he has no input into the abortion decision. He may or may not be consulted by the woman and he finds no support and little counseling available at the clinic. He has no defined role or guidelines to follow, so he becomes frustrated and isolated.

Self-reliance/autonomy

Men are finding it increasingly difficult to act strongly, independently, and self-reliantly in today's society. Their professions are affected more and more by computerization and foreign trade powers. Even the American farmer, who is the epitome of self-reliance, has fallen victim to today's technology and politics. Abortion is yet another area where the male's self-reliance is erased. Under the law, his sexual partner is provided absolute autonomy and he is not allowed to demonstrate his independence or strength.

Even though James wanted to prevent Kathy's abortion, his discomfort over the situation is shown in his words that he didn't know how to go about stopping it. To him, the abortion clinic represented a building of confusion where he had no role or power.

Achievement/success

The expectation that men will achieve is a heavy burden, whether it be in business, pleasure, or personal relationships. When pregnancy and abortion take place in an unmarried relationship, that relationship is likely to fail.

Studies have shown that failure in relationships can lead to alcoholism, suicide, depression, mental illness, physical illness, and premature death. In addition, the male is likely to have greater adjustment problems to abortion the more he asserts himself in the typical aggressive male role. If he objects to the abortion but does not express his feelings, then he will experience a lack of achievement because he wants to provide for the mother and child but is not allowed to.

The only time that abortion supports the male's need to achieve or be successful is in circumstances where the male maintains his self-esteem through sexual achievement. His ability to love is limited and he has little emotional involvement with the woman. Once he has achieved a sexual relationship and possibly pregnancy, he will likely lose interest in her and leave her.

Responsibility/protectiveness

The word *fatherhood* represents a man's ability to provide for and protect his family. It includes not only financial responsibility, but resolving emotional conflicts, directing the family's goals and moral development, and being in command in a crisis. But the man in an abortion situation is not allowed by law to protect his own child. He isn't even allowed to be a part of the abortion decision. He thus cannot fulfill his protective role.

The man who is involved in the abortion decision experiences another type of role strain. While he might desire to protect his own child, he must sacrifice that life for the mother and himself, usually for reasons that affect their quality of life (career, education, inconvenience of pregnancy, etc.).[4]

James felt responsible for the life of his child, but he also felt a strong responsibility to support his wife's decision to have the abortion. Financially, they weren't ready to start a family, and they wanted more time together before they were tied down with the responsibility of raising children. "It would have been a hardship on

---

[4]Ibid., p. 104.

both of us if I had objected to the abortion. I guess I went along with what she wanted, because she wasn't ready to have children," he said.

Men who are expected to be in control and responsible for their actions suddenly find themselves out of control in an abortion situation. Because there is no defined set of guidelines for the male, the father may fulfill the idea that men have no emotions. He won't express what he really feels when the woman goes to the clinic to abort his child. He is concerned about her health and agrees to her wish for abortion only because he has no recourse.

Understanding men's emotional energy

Clinical experience reveals that men become angry when they are not part of a decision-making process and thus feel deceived and manipulated.[5] Their resultant rage is really the frustration of powerlessness, of having no control. Guilt over their role in the pregnancy and their inability to change things without pain is also prevalent.

The rage that a man may feel over his lack of control in an abortion situation is usually blocked because he has not been taught how to experience anger safely. His knowledge that he has no rights in this issue causes him to believe he has no right to be angry. But the man whose child is being aborted needs to unblock the anger he feels before it grows to damaging proportions.

Although the man may not allow his anger and frustration to surface at the time of the abortion, eventually he will deal with it through a process called hooking.[6]

---

[5]Dr. Vincent M. Rue, *Forgotten Fathers: Men and Abortion* (1986), pamphlet produced by Life Cycle Books, P.O. Box 792, Lewiston, NY 14092–0792.

[6]Dr. Jane Steinhauser, "Abortion's Impact on the Father and Familial Relationships," presented at Healing Visions II, the Second National Conference on Post Abortion Counseling, University of Notre Dame (July 20, 1987), available on cassette tape.

This occurs when someone or something triggers a response to his unfinished emotional cycle, and he finds himself reacting to his own emotions and not to the present situation.

Weeks, months, or even years after the abortion, he finds himself in a situation where he explodes over someone else's abortion or another man's frustration over abortion. It appears as though he is reacting to that person's experience, but he is actually reacting to his own unexpressed anger. Thus, he deals with his own abortion issue when he gets "hooked" on another person's experience.

Relationship with partner affected

The emotions men experience as a result of abortion will affect their relationship with the mother of the child. One study found that of the more than 400 couples who went through the abortion experience, 70% of the relationships failed within one month after the abortion.[7] In a second survey by Shostak of 72 men, long after their abortion clinic experience, 25% of the men blamed the abortion for contributing to the end of the relationship.[8] And in interviews with 30 women who had experienced one or more abortions, 46% of the subjects reported a termination of the relationship with the male partner.[9]

Even in those situations where the partners are married, if they disagree over the abortion, their relationship becomes filled with dishonesty, denial, and inequality in marital decision making. Or, they may never talk about the abortion, which lies at the base of the future they build

[7]Rue, op. cit.
[8]Arthur B. Shostak and Gary McLouth with Lynn Seng, *Men and Abortion: Lessons, Losses, and Love* (New York, N.Y.: Praeger Publishers, 1984), p. 105.
[9]Dr. Anne Speckhard, "The Psycho-Social Aspects of Stress Following Abortion," Doctoral Thesis submitted to the University of Minnesota (May 1985), p. 86.

together. Years pass and bitterness grows on both sides. Subconsciously the woman asks herself, what kind of a man is he to let me abort his child? At the same time, he questions why he married a woman who killed her baby.[10] And so their marriage lacks the closeness and honesty that they once enjoyed before the abortion created a void that can never be filled.

What does the male really feel?

When the male is first informed of the unplanned pregnancy, he is naturally shocked. While he may need to express his own feelings of helplessness and frustration, he recognizes that the woman is in an emotional state where he needs to be a supporter. So he will repress his own deep and unexpected feelings. An example is the following male's account:[11]

"I realized it was partly my responsibility, and to that degree I wanted to be responsible about it. But what I also saw from the start was that she was not prepared to handle this any more than anyone else. That enabled me to put my own feelings aside. I did not afford myself the luxury of sitting around and determining how I felt about the abortion. The thing was to keep her alive and going through all of this."

In effect, the male assumes the role of a "solicitous supporter" by reassuring the woman that her needs and wishes are most important. "It was one of the only times in my life when I realized I was involved, but I didn't have the ultimate say. I wasn't really in favor of it at the time,

---

[10]Dr. Jean Garton, "Pastoral Counseling in Crisis: Abortion," presented to counseling class at Concordia Seminary, Ft. Wayne, IN (February 16, 1983), p. 12.
[11]Shostak and McLouth, op. cit., p. 40.

but I realized it was . . . a woman's decision."[12]

By reassuring the woman of his love and support, the male needs to feel that he is collaborating on the steps that need to be taken to protect the woman. Underlying this reaction is the need to do the manly thing. Shostak found that waiting-room males explained their need to win approval from their lover and close friends by doing what was expected of them as the father. Of those 1,000 men surveyed, 42% offered to marry the woman and keep the baby and 25% offered to provide child support if the woman preferred single motherhood. Most of the men offered to pay all the costs of an abortion.[13]

While men attempt to be supportive, many question abortion's morality. Of the 1,000 men surveyed by Shostak, 39% believed life began at conception or when the nervous system began to function. And 26% believed that the procedure taking place as they completed the survey questions was the "killing of a child."[14]

So while the male appears to be supportive of the abortion, what he is actually feeling might include:[15]

- fear of the health hazards of the woman;
- guilt over not preventing the pregnancy;
- anxiety over the possibility that the woman will blame him for having to resort to abortion;
- self-doubt as to his own worth and ability to handle a crisis;
- sadness over the loss of the child, over changes in the relationship, and over the whole abortion experience.

---

[12]Arthur B. Shostak, "Abortion as Fatherhood Glimpsed: Clinic Waiting Room Males as (Former) Expectant Fathers," presented to Eastern Sociological Society Meeting, Philadelphia, PA (March 1985), p. 4.

[13]Ibid., p. 4.

[14]Ibid., p. 7.

[15]Shostak and McLouth, op. cit., p. 41.

Fatherhood lost

Of Shostak's 1,000 waiting-room males, 47% expected emotional and mental problems to develop for them as a result of their abortion experience. Another 39% were uncertain about the possibility.[16] Despite their need to be a supporter of the woman's right to an abortion, 52% of the men had occasional thoughts about the child on the abortion day. Another sample of 75 men who were interviewed months and years after their abortion experience showed that 60% had occasional thoughts of the child. So their involvement with the abortion did not fade with time.[17]

Shostak concluded that males grieve the loss of paternity in a hidden and denied fashion. By seeing the need to reassure the woman of their love and support, the men exhibited strength and relief to cover up their own sorrow. "I only let on what I felt she could handle; I never let her know what I was really feeling."[18]

How a man can cope with guilt and grief

Despite his willingness to support the abortion, afterward a man is as likely to suffer from guilt and grief as the woman. He has lost a child, yet the memory of the unborn child remains as proof of his virility. There are specific things he can do to ease the pain:[19]

First, he can talk about the abortion with the woman, a close friend, counselor or pastor. Talking about it will enable him to admit that it really happened and he was a part of it. If there is a post-abortion support group in his area, he can call and talk to one of the counselors. Some

---

[16]Shostak, op. cit., p. 8.
[17]Ibid., p. 10.
[18]Ibid., p. 10.
[19]Rue, op. cit.

of the groups have male volunteers who have experienced abortion and can understand the feelings of frustration and guilt (see Appendix C).

Second, he needs to acknowledge that he has much unfinished emotional business tied to the abortion. He can stop pretending that it didn't bother him and acknowledge his true feelings about the whole situation. By allowing his feelings to surface, he will gain a greater knowledge of himself and his attitudes toward life and responsibilities. This release will bring with it a self-acceptance and self-identity.

Third, to reconcile the death of his unborn child, he will need to forgive, both himself and the other people involved in the abortion. He will be able to do this only by allowing the truth of the situation to surface, along with his emotions. Before he attempts to forgive others, however, he needs to accept his own feelings about the abortion. If he would like assistance with his healing, he should contact a Christian counselor who can lead him through the healing steps.

James found relief from his guilt over the abortion of his first child only after he became a Christian and learned that he could be forgiven for his sin. "We knew what we had done was wrong, but we didn't realize how wrong until we were saved," James said. "We had never considered the spiritual aspect of abortion until then. When we realized we had taken a life God had created, we cried and asked God to forgive us." James feels that he learned the hard way that life is sacred and a gift from God.

While he has never publicly shared his experience and won't voluntarily admit that his child was aborted, he feels compelled to discourage other people from having abortions. "I tell them abortion is wrong, that it's a human being inside of them."

James has learned from his abortion experience and vows to never repeat it. "Once you realize you made a mistake, you should own up to it and make corrections in your life so that it will never happen again."

THE CHILDREN

Five-year-old Kevin is obsessed with death, not the death of his own immediate family, but with other people. He wants to know if someone is going to die, and when they will die. When he plays with his space creatures, most of them die in combat.

While this may be normal behavior for a five-year-old, Kevin's mom is concerned because he knows that she had an abortion before he was born and he understands that it was a bad thing for her to do. "I do a lot of public speaking about my experience and counsel PAS sufferers over the phone, so he began to question what I was doing. I thought it best to explain to him about the abortion in my life, but lately I've noticed how intrigued he is with death. He never talks about why I aborted his brother or sister, but he seems to want to find out as much as possible about death."

Kevin is one member of another group of people greatly affected by abortion: the children. These are the infants who survive an abortion attempt, siblings of the aborted child, and, really, any child who is born. They are all survivors of the womb, where no legal protection is available for the occupant.

Which children are psychologically affected?

According to psychologists, the degree to which abortion survivors are affected psychologically is determined in part by whether they are aware of the experience, know of siblings who did not survive, or understand society's attitude toward children (that is, that they have value only if they are wanted).[20]

Many children are aware that they exist only because they were chosen. The phrase "wanted child" is common and serves as the basis for keeping or terminating a pregnancy. As a result, children feel secure only when they are pleasing their parents. If there is a family crisis or disagreement, the children will likely blame themselves. "Consequently," said psychiatrist Philip Ney, "a large number of children become overanxious parent pleasers until they can no longer cope. Then they become self-blaming and depressed or hostile and rebellious. Though parents may fail to recognize the child's depression because of their own preoccupation with guilt, there is an increasing incidence of depression and suicide among children that may be partly explained by this mechanism."[21]

The survivor syndrome

Children who are siblings of the aborted child may experience what is called the survivor syndrome. These children feel guilty for surviving, which, in turn, produces depression. The depression may show up as irritability and lethargy, which the parents often interpret as rudeness and disrespect. Also, the children are angry toward their parents, but take it out on younger siblings, which causes the parents to be angry. The child may intentionally bring on the parents' wrath because he feels that he

[20]Dr. Philip G. Ney, "A Consideration of Abortion Survivors," *Child Psychiatry and Human Development* (Vol. 13–3, Spring 1983), p. 168.
[21]Ibid., pp. 171–172.

should be punished for surviving.[22] The child wonders, subconsciously or consciously, "Why was I allowed to live when my brother or sister was killed?"

Types of survivors

According to Ney, children can be classified according to three types of abortion survivors:[23]

The *haunted child* lives in distrust of his future because he knows there was an abortion by his parents but he doesn't know the details. He is haunted by the mystery of it all and is afraid to ask for details and why it happened for fear of discovering something more awful than he already imagines.

Mark knows his parents aborted their first child because they talk about their experience when they speak at pro-life seminars. Six-year-old Mark understands that abortion is wrong and that it killed his older brother or sister. But he is afraid to ask his parents why they allowed this awful thing to happen. Don't they really love children? If they didn't want children, why didn't they kill him, too?

The *bound child* is one whose parents attempt to control the factors that led to the abortion. These factors might include social pressure, economic necessity, or convenience. They want to make sure it never happens again, so they overprotect the surviving child against any perceived hostilities. The result is a repression of the child's intelligence, adaptability and curiosity.

Elizabeth's parents had an abortion before they were

[22]Dr. Philip G. Ney, "Infant Abortion and Child Abuse: Cause and Effect," *The Psychological Aspects of Abortion* (Washington, D.C.: University Publications of America, Inc., 1979), pp. 29–30.
[23]Dr. Philip G. Ney, "A Consideration of Abortion Survivors," *Child Psychiatry and Human Development* (Vol. 13–3, Spring 1983), p. 171.

married and still college students. They wanted to wait to start their family after they had graduated, married and settled with jobs and a home. After Elizabeth was born, her mother decided to stay home with her because she didn't trust someone else to look after her baby. Now four years old, Elizabeth is not allowed to play with any neighbor children because her mother is afraid she will catch colds and other childhood diseases from them. The only children she plays with are her two cousins who live 30 miles away. Her mother, believing she must be Elizabeth's primary educator, is considering teaching her at home so she won't be exposed to the influences of other children and adults at public school.

The *substitute child* is an especially wanted child who was conceived to replace the aborted child. This child carries his parents' high expectations, which he may not be able to fulfill. If he does fail, his parents overreact and feel let down by this child in whom they had placed all their hopes and dreams.

Age 15, Kevin is a promising wrestler for his high school squad and an honor student. His father had been a state wrestling champion in high school and expected Kevin to follow in his footsteps. What Kevin doesn't realize is that his parents aborted an older brother at four months into the pregnancy when they were high school seniors. They couldn't get married because his father would risk losing his wrestling scholarship to the state university. So they had aborted the baby after weeks of struggling with their dilemma. His father went on to wrestle for the university but lost his scholarship in his second year. In his frustration and disappointment, he dropped out of school and married Kevin's mother, who had waited patiently for him. They settled in their hometown where he went to work in the family business. Two years later Kevin was born and his father began to dream of wrestling medals and tournaments that he should have won and that his first, aborted son could have won.

Abortion and child abuse

While a popular pro-abortion argument says that unwanted, unaborted babies will be victims of increased child abuse, studies indicate that child abuse is more frequent among mothers who have previously had an abortion. The reason is that the guilt from the abortion causes depression, which hinders the mother's ability to bond with future children.[24] The depression may not surface until the birth of the subsequent child, when the unresolved grief for the first child appears. Mourning will be more difficult when the mother has desired or contributed to the death of the lost baby. Her inability to bond with future children results in a greater chance of abuse and neglect.[25]

When Julie, a senior in high school, discovered she was pregnant, she felt that abortion was her only choice. She wanted to graduate and go on to college, not marry and have a baby, so she had the child aborted. She did attend college for two quarters but quit to work when she ran out of money. Soon after quitting college, Julie learned that she was again pregnant. This time she married the father and had the baby, born two years after her abortion.

Julie loves her daughter, now three years old, but for most of the first year of her life, Julie felt ambivalence toward her little girl. "I kept imagining I should have another child running round. I almost felt hostility toward Jessie, because she wasn't perfect. She was a difficult, col-

---

[24]Ibid., p. 172.
[25]Ibid., p. 173.

icky infant and a difficult toddler. I guess I expected her to fill the spot of the first child. Mostly I had a feeling that another child should be there. I wasn't able to feel close to Jessie because I always visualized another child two steps up."

This difficulty in bonding with subsequent children is the result of the rationalization process the parents used in order to abort their first child. To abort their child, they had to take away his human qualities and deny his dependency on them, his need for protection and care. This diminishes their ability to understand their subsequent newborn baby and to respond to his needs.

Men especially are subject to difficulties in bonding with future children. The man who has gone through a prior abortion experience is likely to remain aloof about the developing child until after the baby's birth. Even then, his concern may be less than normal because of his hesitation to become emotionally involved and risk being hurt.[26]

Having an abortion may decrease a male or female's natural restraint against an occasional feeling of rage felt toward a small child dependent on their care.[27] Normally a signal of distress from a child will cause the parent to find out what the problem is and take care of it. A parent overcomes her natural impulse to care for a child's helplessness when she chooses abortion. That same impulse is thus weakened when dealing with subsequent pregnancies and children. After having suppressed the preserving instinct once before with the aborted child, the suppressed response may become less effective in holding back rage against the helplessness of a newborn or the

---

[26]Ibid., p. 173.
[27]Dr. Philip G. Ney, "Relationship Between Abortion and Child Abuse," *Canadian Journal of Psychiatry* (November 1979), pp. 611- 612.

crying of a toddler or the questions of the preschooler. This might explain why people who are beaten or neglected as a child will respond to cries of distress with rage or neglect.[28]

Abortion's other effects on children

Increased hostility

As adults weigh the cost of raising a child against the material goods they desire, they consider the increasing demands of the younger generation. To the parents, it appears that the younger generation always wants more. To the youth, it seems that their parents don't care enough about them to give them time and love but only material goods. The threatened adults may retaliate with aggression, including physical and emotional battering.[29]

Suicide

For the child who survived abortion, the unsuccessful abortion attempt can be unconsciously remembered and he may attempt to duplicate it by repeated, unsuccessful suicide attempts.[30] The child is actually compulsively acting out a memory, and what may be interpreted as insanity is actually a memory. Once the connection is made between the two events, the child, most likely now a grown person, is relieved of having to repeat the abortion attempt through suicide.

---

[28]Ibid., p. 612.

[29]Ibid., p. 613.

[30]Dr. Andrew Feldmar, "The Embryology of Consciousness: What is a Normal Pregnancy?" *The Psychological Aspects of Abortion* (Washington, D.C.: University Publications of America, Inc., 1979), p. 21.

Diminishing value of children

The value of children has diminished as the number of abortions has increased. More and more people would rather not have any children. As Ney said, "Logically, when people stop wanting a child, it loses value. If the unborn child has no value and it is permissible to kill it, then it is defensible to kill children who have lost value because they are not wanted. . . . People do not harm what they value highly. As children lose in worth, it becomes easier to neglect or dispose of them. Besides, both those who abort children and those who murder them say they do it 'out of love.' "[31]

How to fight negative side effects of abortion

Parents who want to combat these negative side effects of abortion can do so by first examining where they are in their own healing process. Are they still living with the guilt of the abortion or have they admitted their guilt, asked God for forgiveness, and forgiven others involved in their abortion decision and themselves? They need to have advanced through each of the healing steps described in the earlier chapters before concentrating on healing the relationships with their children.

If they believe they are emotionally healed from their abortion experience, or are in the final stages of healing, they should next look at their relationship with each of their surviving children. They need to evaluate their feelings for each child and how they treat him. Does the child make them angry for no apparent reason? Do they feel anxious whenever the child is out of sight? How do they regard their role as parents? Do they feel comfortable or inadequate in this role?

---

[31]Ney, op. cit., p. 613.

Have they told the child or children about their abortion? How was this done—in anger or in a loving manner? How did the child react?

If they haven't told the child about the abortion, do they suspect that the child knows anyway?

As the parent considers these questions, they may discover that the relationship is less than desirable and want to make some changes. They should seek the help of a professional Christian counselor, who can recommend specific steps to follow.

Before contacting a counselor, parents can do a few things on their own. First, they should be honest about the abortion, especially if the child knows or suspects that it occurred. They should be willing to discuss why it happened and admit that they made a mistake. If they feel comfortable writing, they might try expressing their thoughts on paper, either as a letter to the child, or to clarify thoughts for themselves. Discussion of the thoughts can follow. Parents should be honest about what happened and willing to answer any questions the child might ask.

Second, parents should work at building a better relationship with the child by spending more time with him, whether it's helping him with his homework, taking him to the park, or reading a story together. If the child is a teenager, they can go camping or shopping together, build a project they both enjoy working on, or just sit and talk to each other. If the child is grown and living away from home, they can write letters or frequently call him on the phone. If possible, they should arrange short visits, when all the family members can spend time together. The ultimate goal, no matter what the age of the child, is to build a good relationship by spending time with each other.

Throughout all their efforts at building meaningful relationships with their children, parents should make use of a powerful tool available to them as Christians: prayer. Through daily prayer, they can ask for and expect to receive God's guidance in rebuilding their family life. "And my God will meet all your needs according to his glorious riches in Christ Jesus" (Phil. 4:19).

Appendix A

SCRIPTURE

(All verses taken from the New International Version of The Holy Bible)

Love replaces self-condemnation

"Forget the former things; do not dwell on the past. See, I am doing a new thing! Now it springs up; do you not perceive it? I am making a way in the desert and streams in the wasteland" (Isa. 43:18–19).

"Comfort, comfort my people, says your God. Speak tenderly to Jerusalem, and proclaim to her that her hard service has been completed, that her sin has been paid for, that she has received from the Lord's hand double for all her sins" (Isa. 40:1–2).

"Brothers, I do not consider myself yet to have taken hold of it. But one thing I do: Forgetting what is behind and straining toward what is ahead, I press on toward the goal to win the prize for which God has called me heavenward in Christ Jesus" (Phil. 3:13–14).

"For everything that was written in the past was written to teach us, so that through endurance and the encouragement of the Scriptures we might have hope" (Rom. 15:4).

Trade guilt for joy

"You turned my wailing into dancing; you removed my sackcloth and clothed me with joy, that my heart may sing to you and not be silent. O Lord my God, I will give you thanks forever" (Ps. 30:11–12).

"The Lord has done great things for us, and we are filled with joy" (Ps. 126:3).

"Rejoice with those who rejoice; mourn with those who mourn" (Rom. 12:15).

"Until now you have not asked for anything in my name. Ask and you will receive, and your joy will be complete" (John 16:24).

"As the Father has loved me, so have I loved you. Now remain in my love. If you obey my commands, you will remain in my love, just as I have obeyed my Father's commands and remain in his love. I have told you this so that my joy may be in you and that your joy may be complete" (John 15:9–11).

"If you have any encouragement from being united with Christ, if any comfort from his love, if any fellowship with the Spirit, if any tenderness and compassion, then make my joy complete by being like-minded, having the same love, being one in spirit and purpose" (Phil. 2:1–2).

A present hope

"He will wipe every tear from their eyes. There will be no more death or mourning or crying or pain, for the old order of things has passed away" (Rev. 21:4).

"For the Lamb at the center of the throne will be their shepherd; he will lead them to springs of living water.

And God will wipe away every tear from their eyes" (Rev. 7:17).

"Blessed are those who mourn, for they will be comforted" (Matt. 5:4).

"And for this we labor and strive, that we have put our hope in the living God, who is the Savior of all men, and especially of those who believe" (1 Tim. 4:10).

"This is what the Lord says: 'A voice is heard in Ramah, mourning and great weeping, Rachel weeping for her children and refusing to be comforted, because her children are no more.' This is what the Lord says: 'Restrain your voice from weeping and your eyes from tears, for your work will be rewarded,' declares the Lord. 'They will return from the land of the enemy. So there is hope for your future,' declares the Lord. 'Your children will return to their own land' " (Jer. 31:15–17).

Called to serve

"Therefore, if anyone is in Christ, he is a new creation; the old has gone, the new has come. All this is from God, who reconciled us to himself through Christ and gave us the ministry of reconciliation: that God was reconciling the world to himself in Christ, not counting men's sins against them. And he has committed to us the message of reconciliation" (2 Cor. 5:17–19).

"Praise be to the God and Father of our Lord Jesus Christ, the Father of compassion and the God of all comfort, who comforts us in all our troubles, so that we can comfort those in any trouble with the comfort we ourselves have received from God" (2 Cor. 1:3–4).

NINE STEPS FOR PERSONAL GROWTH*

Step One: I recognize that I am powerless to heal the damage my abortion has created in my life. I look to Jesus Christ for the power to make me whole.

Step Two: I will be willing to share my feelings with at least one other person to release myself from the secrecy and shame and allow my healing to begin.

Step Three: I understand the shame, guilt and emotional distress I suffer is a consequence of my actions. I will acknowledge these feelings and seek to resolve them.

Step Four: I will choose to accept mourning as a part of the healing process as I grieve the loss of my child. I will work through the different stages of grief with the help of God.

Step Five: I am willing to confess to God that I alone am accountable to Him for the loss of my child. I cannot hold resentment toward others who have assisted or

---

*Used by permission from Conquerors Post Abortion Support Group, 3361 Republic Avenue, Suite 201, Minneapolis, MN 55426. Telephone: (612) 920–8117

pushed me into that decision.

Step Six: I accept responsibility for the loss of my child through abortion, but I will choose to forgive myself and others and I will accept Christ's forgiveness.

Step Seven: I acknowledge that I am an important person and I am special in God's sight. With His help, I will develop a positive self-image and work toward my full potential.

Step Eight: With the help of God, I will use my experience to protect and save the lives of other mothers and babies and will help other women who have had abortions.

Step Nine: I acknowledge God's sovereignty and I will strive to learn His plan for my life. I will choose to continue the process of healing from my abortion experience until that healing is complete, regardless of the pain and sorrow that those memories might bring to the surface.

APPENDIX C

POST-ABORTION SUPPORT GROUPS

The following groups will provide post-abortion counseling, either by professional or volunteer counselors. The national offices are noted with an asterisk if the organization has representatives in various states. Contact the national office for the address and telephone number of the office nearest you.

American Victims of Abortion *
Suite 402
419 7th St. NW
Washington, DC 20004
(202) 626–8800

Open Arms *
P.O. Box 7188
Federal Way, WA 98003
(206) 839–8919

PACE (Post Abortion Counseling and Education) *
701 W. Broad St.
Suite 405
Falls Church, VA 22046

or
P.O. Box 35032
Tucson, AZ 85740
(602) 742–5835

WEBA (Women Exploited By Abortion) *
151 River Ave.
Eugene, Oregon 97404

International, National, State and Local Women Exploited by Abortion minister to hurting women throughout the world. Members of this organization have gone through the abortion experience, have found healing in Jesus Christ, and are prepared to counsel those in need of restoration.

After Abortion Helpline
P.O. Box 28633
21 Violet Street
Providence, RI 02908
(401) 941–3050

Archdiocese of St. Paul-Minneapolis
Post-Abortion Counseling Program
226 Summit Avenue
St. Paul, MN 55102
(612) 291–4424

CARE (Counseling for Abortion Related Experiences)
709B Investment Building
Pittsburgh, PA 15222

Conquerors
New Life Homes & Family Services
3361 Republic Avenue Suite 201
Minneapolis, MN 55426
(612) 920–8117

Come Alive Ministries
101 Peninsula Blvd.
Morgantown, WV 26505
(304) 296–111

Project Rachel
c/o Respect Life Office
Archdiocese of Milwaukee
P.O. Box 2018
Milwaukee, WI 53201
(414) 769–3391

The Puzzle Project
100 S. Elmwood Avenue
Buffalo, NY 14202
(716) 854–5434

RETURN
Joliet Diocesan Life Center
Route 53 & Airport Road
Romeoville, IL 60441
(815) 838–1002

FOR MEN:

Fathers for Life
Fathers' Rights Legal Services Association
3623 Douglas Avenue
Des Moines, IA 50310
(515) 277–8789 or
(515) 233–2750 (evenings and weekends)

Appendix D

ADDITIONAL READING

Banks, Bill and Sue. *Ministering to Abortion's Aftermath.* Kirkwood, MO: Impact Books, Inc., 137 W. Jefferson, Kirkwood, MO 63122. (1982)

Ervin, Paula. *Women Exploited: The Other Victims of Abortion.* Huntington, IN: Our Sunday Visitor, Inc., 200 Noll Plaza, Huntington, IN 46750. (1985)

Koerbel, Pam. *Abortion's Second Victim.* Wheaton, IL: Victor Books, Box 1825, Wheaton, IL 60187. (1986)

Kuenning, Delores. *Helping People Through Grief.* Minneapolis, MN: Bethany House Publishers, 6820 Auto Club Road, Minneapolis, MN 55438. (1987)

Linn, Dennis and Matthew, S.J., and Sheila Fabricant. *At Peace with the Unborn: A Book for Healing.* Mahwah, NJ: Paulist Press, 997 Macarthur Blvd., Mahwah, NJ 07430. (1985)

Mall, David and Walter F. Watts, M.D. *The Psychological Aspects of Abortion.* Washington, D.C.: University Publications of America, Inc. (1979)

Mannion, Michael T. *Abortion & Healing: A Cry to be*

Whole. Kansas City, MO: Sheed and Ward, 115 E. Armour Blvd., P.O. Box 281, Kansas City, MO 64141–0281. Telephone: (800) 821–7926. (1986)

McAll, Kenneth, M.D. *Healing the Family Tree.* London: Sheldon Press, SPCK, Marylebone Road, London NW1 4DU. (1982)

Minirth, Frank B., M.D., and Paul D. Meier, M.D. *Happiness Is a Choice (A Manual on the Symptoms, Causes, and Cures of Depression).* Grand Rapids, MI: Baker Book House Co., Box 6287, Grand Rapids, MI 49506. (1978)

Reardon, David C. *Aborted Women, Silent No More.* Chicago: Loyola University Press, 3441 North Ashland Avenue, Chicago, IL 60657. (1987)

Shostak, Arthur B. and Gary McLouth with Lynn Seng. *Men and Abortion; Lessons, Losses, and Love.* New York: Praeger Publishers, 521 Fifth Avenue, New York, NY 10175. (1984)

Stanford, Susan M., Ph.D. *Will I Cry Tomorrow?* Old Tappan: Fleming H. Revell Co., Central Avenue, Old Tappan, NJ 07675. (1986)

Additional Resources Available From:

National Youth Pro-Life Coalition*
Jackson Avenue
Hastings-on-Hudson
New York, NY 10706
(914) 478–0103

---

*Sponsor of post-abortion counseling, ministry and reconciliation programs.

LINCOLN CHRISTIAN COLLEGE AND SEMINARY